MERENESS'

ESSENTIALS OF PSYCHIATRIC NURSING

Learning & Activity Guide

LANGDALE UNIT/
FORENSIC PSYCHIATRY
SERVICE

MERENESS'

ESSENTIALS OF PSYCHIATRIC NURSING

Learning & Activity Guide

Carol Ruth Lofstedt, RN, MA

Professor of Nursing
Bronx Community College
Bronx, New York

THIRD EDITION

THE C. V. MOSBY COMPANY

St. Louis • Baltimore • Philadelphia • Toronto   1990

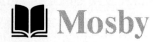

Editor: Linda L. Duncan
Developmental editor: Joanna May
Project manager: Teri Merchant
Designer: Susan E. Lane
Editing and production: CRACOM Corporation

THIRD EDITION

Previous editions copyrighted 1982, 1986

Printed in the United States of America
International Standard Book Number 0-8016-5300-2

The C. V. Mosby Company
11830 Westline Industrial Drive, St. Louis, Missouri 63146

GW/D/D 9 8 7 6 5 4 3 2

Preface

PURPOSE

The third edition of the *Learning and Activity Guide* has been designed with several goals in mind. First, because it articulates section by section, chapter by chapter with the thirteenth edition of *Mereness' Essentials of Psychiatric Nursing* by Cecelia Monat Taylor, this guide provides exercises and activities to enhance and reenforce the learnings set forth in that textbook. Second, the guide is designed to meet the educational needs of the beginning psychiatric nursing student. Third, the guide can also be useful to the graduate nurse who desires to review the theoretical bases for understanding mental health and mental illness, the tools of psychiatric nursing, and the care of emotionally ill individuals. Fourth, because the guide has been developed on the principle that learning occurs best when the student is actively, rather than passively, involved in the learning process, the guide strives to actively involve students in their own learning through the use of a variety of thoughtful and, I hope, interesting and stimulating exercises. Finally, with the increasing national concern that many students today are lacking in their ability to read, write, and communicate effectively, the exercises in the guide have been designed to use the skills of reading, writing, listening, and speaking. Gone are the days when these skills are the sole responsibility of one or two disciplines; it is the responsibility of all educators in all disciplines to reenforce what has been taught by our colleagues in the humanities. All students need multiple opportunities to read their texts, write their thoughts, share orally their ideas and feelings, and listen and respond to the contributions of others. The exercises and activites in the *Learning and Activity Guide* provide opportunities for students to use all these basic skills.

Although the third edition of the *Learning and Activity Guide* could enhance and enrich the learnings in any basic psychiatric nursing textbook, the guide is primarily designed to accompany the thirteenth edition of *Mereness' Essentials of Psychiatric Nursing* by Cecelia Monat Taylor. The guide subscribes to the belief set forth in that textbook that all nurses need a sound theoretical and experiential foundation in order to give purposeful and concerned care to emotionally ill individuals. It also recognizes that knowledge and skills that were once considered unique to psychiatric nursing have relevance to all areas of nursing; beginning level practitioners should be encouraged to use such knowledge and skills in the care of all clients.

DESCRIPTION   Revisions in the third edition of the *Learning and Activity Guide* fall into two categories. First, there are revisions based on changes made in the textbook. Second, there are revisions made in the nature and number of exercises, activities, test items, and word games.

Changes in content and organization of the third edition of the guide reflect the changes in content and organization made in the thirteenth edition of the textbook. There are now five sections and 26 chapters in both books. The content of the sixth section that appeared in the previous edition has not been eliminated. The chapters on legal matters and current issues affecting psychiatric nursing have been revised and moved to Section One, The Context of Psychiatric Nursing Practice, where they help provide a foundation for all the content that follows. The exercises in this section focus the reader on treatment measures used through the centuries, the contemporary community mental health system, and the roles of the interdisciplinary mental health care team. In addition, exercises in this section review client rights and their nursing implications. They also encourage the reader to identify and discuss issues affecting the care of the mentally ill and the current practice and future of psychiatric nursing.

Section Two, The Tools of the Psychiatric Nurse, no longer includes a chapter on psychotropic medications. This content has been essentially incorporated into the discussion on the care of individual clients in Section Four. Chapter 5, Principles of Psychiatric Nursing, has been developed out of material formerly covered in the chapter on self-awareness. Chapter 9, The Nursing Process, continues to provide a sound organizational basis for nursing practice. In addition to the NANDA Approved Nursing Diagnostic Categories (1988), the ANA Classification of Human Responses of Concern for Psychiatric Mental Health Nursing Practice, Draft IV-R (September 20, 1988) has been included in the revised edition of the textbook and the guide. Both formats are used throughout the guide to help the reader develop appropriate nursing diagnoses for individual clients. Several exercises in this section provide opportunities for the reader to achieve greater self-awareness as it applies to mental illness, psychiatric nursing, and the care of mentally ill persons. Other exercises use principles of psychiatric nursing, promote effective patterns of verbal and nonverbal communication, facilitate understanding of nurse-client interactions and the various roles and functions of the nurse, evaluate both the physical and socioemotional factors of the hospital environment, and apply the multiple phases of the nursing process to the care of persons with emotional problems. Clinical situations are introduced at this time to provide interest and reality.

Two new chapters: Chapter 13, Biological Factors Influencing Mental Health and Mental Illness, and Chapter 14, Cultural Factors Influencing Mental Health and Mental Illness, have been included in Section Three, Theoretical Bases for Understanding Mental Health and Mental Illness. The addition of this content in the revised editions of the textbook and the guide reflects the increasing interest in the roles played by both biology and culture in the promotion of mental health and the development of mental illness. Chapter 11, Psychosocial Theories of Personality Development, has been revised significantly to include Piaget's stages of cognitive development. The exercises in this section provide readers with an opportunity to use general systems theory, the theory of stress and adaptation, and the psychosocial theories of Freud, Sullivan, Erikson, and Piaget as they apply to normal personality development. In addition, other exercises focus on the influence of anxiety and stress and biology and culture on mental health and mental illness.

Section Four, The Consumers of Psychiatric Nursing, focuses on adults, adolescents, children, the elderly, and the physically ill whose behavioral patterns have become dysfunctional. This section now includes content on the needs and care of persons with borderline personality disorder in Chapter 20, Individuals with Personality Disorders, of mentally retarded and emotionally ill children in Chapter 22, Populations at Risk: Children and Adolescents, and of individuals with autoimmune deficiency syndrome (AIDS) in Chapter 23, Populations at Risk: The Physically Ill. Exercises in this section use client situations extensively, although not exclusively, to utilize the tools of psychiatric nursing introduced in Section Two and to apply the theories covered in Section Three of the textbook to develop beginning understanding of the nature of various disorders and appropriate nursing care. A major focus is on use of the nursing process in carrying out therapeutic client care. Multiple opportunities to work with both the ANA and NANDA nursing diagnostic frameworks are provided. Exercises focusing on the use of psychotropic medications are included in the care of individuals with thought disorders, mood disorders, and anxiety disorders. A sample drug card format is provided to encourage readers to set up a personal drug file on their individual clients if they have not already done so. The need for continued self-awareness is emphasized throughout the section.

Section Five, Multidisciplinary Psychiatric Interventions, includes the care of persons in a crisis state as well as intervention in groups and in families. Material on the recognition and care of the abused child has been revised and expanded in Chapter 26, Family Theory and Intervention. Exercises in this section help the reader identify the phases and characteristics of a crisis state and provide a review of communication skills in a crisis interview, identify the phases of group development, differentiate between the characteristics of therapeutic and socialization groups, identify the roles individuals assume in group situations, review the nature of families in terms of their functions, dynamics, types, characteristics, and effectiveness.

FORMAT   All chapters of the *Learning and Activity Guide* begin with a brief introduction, contain a statement of purpose, and identify a series of objectives to be achieved by completing the exercises in the chapter. The introductory overview, as well as the narrative that accompanies some of the exercises, emphasizes material covered in the text and occasionally introduces new content. This has been done to create interest, to clarify, and to provide a foundation for exercises requiring additional information. This narrative is meant to supplement and enhance, not replace, the content presented in the textbook. The objectives structure the presentation of the exercises, the content of which follows the content of the text and has been selected for emphasis. Exercises vary in style, scope, and depth throughout the guide. At reader request, the number of case situations has been increased. Although the content of the text and the guide are organized in a logical, sequential fashion, no assumption is made that all the chapters will be read and, if read, will necessarily be read in the order in which they are presented. Therefore no effort has been made to develop exercises that are progressively more difficult in the final sections of the guide.

The third edition of the guide continues to present multiple test items at the end of each chapter, allowing readers to check out their understandings before proceeding to another chapter. All items have been reviewed and revised to reflect changes in the textbook. Many new items have been added, and the total number of items in each chapter has been increased.

Each of the five sections concludes with several word games and section exercises. Persons familiar with word puzzles will probably recognize most of these types of games, even though some of the names may be unfamiliar, and some variations may exist in the form. Word Search and Cross Hatch word games provide readers with an opportunity to familiarize themselves with vocabulary used in the respective sections; Fill-Ins involve the defining of specific terms; Quote-a-Crostics test and reenforce content in a specific section and at the same time introduce the readers to pertinent quotations from fictional or nonfictional works. Once the Quote-a-Crostics are solved, the quotation, its source, and its author will be revealed, and the reader may be encouraged to read further in these works. Logic Problems provide opportunities to use problem-solving techniques inherent in the nursing process. Added to the third edition of the guide are several matching exercises that primarily review the contributions made by leaders to the fields of psychiatry and psychiatric nursing.

In addition to the answers to the test items and solutions to the word games and section exercises, the Appendix contains suggested responses to the chapter activities and exercises. These were added to the second edition of the guide at the request of readers. However, I continue to advocate that the text be read first and the exercises completed next, either independently or discussed in small groups. Finally, the reader's responses can then be compared with the responses in the Appendix and discrepancies checked out with the textbook.

The Index has been completely revised and updated. It primarily identifies the content of the exercises in the chapters and should be helpful to anyone who wishes additional practice in selected areas that are threaded throughout the guide, such as communication skills, nursing process, nursing action, and self-awareness.

I wish to acknowledge all the friends, family members, and colleagues who expressed interest in the progress of the manuscript. Special thanks are extended to my friend and colleague, Dr. J. Mae Pepper, Professor and Chairperson, Department of Nursing, Mercy College, Dobbs Ferry, New York, for her encouragement and support throughout various stages of the development of the manuscript.

Carol Ruth Lofstedt

Contents

MERENESS'

ESSENTIALS OF PSYCHIATRIC NURSING
Learning & Activity Guide

1

The mental health delivery system and health care team

INTRODUCTION

"This chapter traces the treatment of mentally ill individuals from prehistoric times to the present in the belief that an appreciation of the history of the treatment of mentally ill persons can aid in understanding the contemporary system of mental health delivery."*

Although mentally ill persons have sometimes been revered and treated with sympathy, acceptance, and compassion, more often than not they have been misunderstood, rejected, and exploited. In prehistoric times, for example, tribal rites were commonly used in an effort to alter bizarre behavior. In the early Greek and Roman eras, as well as during the Middle Ages, both humane and harsh treatments were carried out. During the sixteenth and seventeenth centuries mentally ill persons were often imprisoned and displayed for public ridicule. It was not until the eighteenth and nineteenth centuries that political and social reforms began to impact on their care in a positive way.

In the United States, prior to the American Civil War, moral treatment was popular in certain sections of the country. It emphasized humane, individualized care of mentally ill individuals in homelike surroundings. But as the number of persons requiring care for mental problems increased, moral treatment was replaced by custodial care. Although custodial care provided a protective environment for the control of deviant behaviors that were disrupting and disturbing to the families of mentally ill persons and to the communities from which they came, treatment was not a major priority. Mental illness was viewed as a stigma, and mentally ill people were again perceived as sources of embarrassment and persons to be hidden away and forgotten. Large mental institutions, some housing thousands of persons, grew up. They were often located in remote, rural areas, and little effort was made to help hospitalized persons and their families maintain ties. The phenomenon of institutionalization was prevalent as isolation from family and community encouraged hospitalized individuals to adapt to and accept the role of patient and resist efforts to be returned to the community.

*From Taylor CM: Mereness' essentials of psychiatric nursing, ed 13, St Louis, 1990, The CV Mosby Co, chap 1.

Four events contributed significantly to a change in the care of mentally ill people as we know it today: the development of the health care professions, the introduction of the therapeutic community concept, the discovery and use of psychotropic medications, and the evolution of the community mental health movement. During the last half of the nineteenth century four health care professions—psychiatric nursing, psychiatry, clinical psychology, and psychiatric social work—began to emerge and today make up the core mental health team. In the 1950s the therapeutic community concept, which provided hospitalized individuals with an opportunity to achieve a more constructive social adjustment, was introduced from England. Also at this time psychotropic agents, particularly the antipsychotic medications, were discovered. Hospitalized persons who were once thought to be hopeless responded to these medications. The medications helped them control their behavior and become more receptive to other treatment modalities, including milieu therapy and the "talking therapies" carried out by the members of the mental health team. The use of medications also facilitated the return of hospitalized individuals to the community and helped reduce the population in mental hospitals. These events probably paved the way for the community mental health movement of the 1960s and played a major role in the deinstitutionalization of many mentally ill people.

The exercises in this chapter are designed to help you better understand the interdisciplinary mental health care team, the contemporary mental health system within which it functions, and the historical background from which they both evolved.

OBJECTIVES

1. To identify the attitudes and treatment methods to which mentally ill people have been exposed from prehistoric times to the current day.
2. To list the general goals of a comprehensive community mental health program.
3. To describe the similarities in practice existing among all community mental health care centers.
4. To identify the roles and functions of the members of the mental health team.

EXERCISES

1 From prehistoric times to the present day, mentally ill persons have been exposed to a wide variety of attitudes and treatment methods, not all of which have been therapeutic. Listed below are twenty activities and seven eras in history. Identify the era in which each activity predominated by placing a check in the box in the appropriate column. The first one has been filled in to help you get started.

Activities		Eras in history						
		Prehistoric	Greek-Roman	Middle ages	16-17th centuries	18th century	19th century	20th century
Mentally ill individuals were:								
1. Treated with tribal rites.		☑	☐	☐	☐	☐	☐	☐
2. Abandoned in the wilderness and left to die.		☐	☐	☐	☐	☐	☐	☐
3. Exposed to fresh air, sunshine, and diverting activities.		☐	☐	☐	☐	☐	☐	☐
4. Purged, bled, whipped, starved, and chained.		☐	☐	☐	☐	☐	☐	☐
5. Exorcised of evil spirits by the laying on of hands.		☐	☐	☐	☐	☐	☐	☐
6. Confined in jails, dungeons, and almshouses.		☐	☐	☐	☐	☐	☐	☐
7. Exhibited to the public for ridicule and profit.		☐	☐	☐	☐	☐	☐	☐
8. Released from confinement in chains.		☐	☐	☐	☐	☐	☐	☐
9. Restrained in inhumane devices called tranquilizers.		☐	☐	☐	☐	☐	☐	☐
10. Relegated to the poorhouse and sold at auction.		☐	☐	☐	☐	☐	☐	☐
11. Housed in large, remote, self-supporting institutions.		☐	☐	☐	☐	☐	☐	☐
12. Provided with custodial care.		☐	☐	☐	☐	☐	☐	☐
13. Exploited as free labor in state institutions.		☐	☐	☐	☐	☐	☐	☐
14. Introduced to the treatment techniques of S. Freud.		☐	☐	☐	☐	☐	☐	☐
15. Exposed to reforms following the mental hygiene movement.		☐	☐	☐	☐	☐	☐	☐
16. Administered psychotropic agents.		☐	☐	☐	☐	☐	☐	☐
17. Exposed to milieu therapy and open-door policies.		☐	☐	☐	☐	☐	☐	☐
18. Cared for in community mental health centers.		☐	☐	☐	☐	☐	☐	☐
19. Treated with crisis-oriented therapy.		☐	☐	☐	☐	☐	☐	☐
20. Cared for by an interdisciplinary mental health team.		☐	☐	☐	☐	☐	☐	☐

2 List four general goals of a comprehensive community mental health program.

1. _____

2. _____

3. _____

4. _____

3 To achieve these goals, community mental health centers follow six similar practices. List these practices. The first one has been filled in to help you get started.

   1. Provide comprehensive and continuous service to the consumer.
   2.
   3.
   4.
   5.
   6.

4 Listed below are ten roles and functions of the members of the interdisciplinary health team, with the exception of the psychiatric nurse, whose roles and functions will be covered in Chapter 6. Identify which roles/functions are primarily associated with which team member by placing a check in the box in the appropriate column. The first one has been filled in to help you get started.

Roles and functions	Team members			
	Clinical psychologist	Psychiatric social worker	Psychiatrist	Activity therapist
1. Strives to meet both physical and emotional needs.	☐	☐	☑	☐
2. Prescribes medications and carries out somatic treatments.	☐	☐	☐	☐
3. Assesses familial, social, and environmental background.	☐	☐	☐	☐
4. Provides tools that promote nonverbal communication.	☐	☐	☐	☐
5. Makes a medical diagnosis.	☐	☐	☐	☐
6. Administers and interprets projective techniques to make a psychiatric diagnosis.	☐	☐	☐	☐
7. Provides work and/or recreational experiences.	☐	☐	☐	☐
8. Plans and implements follow-up care.	☐	☐	☐	☐
9. Emphasizes the concept of object relations in planning programs.	☐	☐	☐	☐
10. Engages in research and scholarly study of human behavior.	☐	☐	☐	☐

TEST ITEMS

DIRECTIONS: Select the *best* response. (Answers appear in the Appendix.)

1 Mental health care during the early Greek era was primarily carried out in the:

   a Family.   c Almshouse.
   b Temple.   d Prison.

2 The technique of "exorcising" evil spirits and demons from mentally ill persons as performed by holy men consisted of:

   a Laying on of hands.   c Whipping.
   b Burning at the stake.   d Bleeding.

3 Gheel, Belgium is *best* known as the:
   a Birthplace of St. Dymphna, the patron saint of the mentally ill.
   b Location of "Bedlam," a notorious lunatic asylum in the sixteenth century.
   c City where the first psychiatric institution was built.
   d Site of the first community-based center for the care of mentally ill individuals.

4 In the matter of reforms for the treatment of mental illness, Philippe Pinel was to France as the brothers Tuke were to:
   a Belgium.   c Germany.
   b Switzerland.   d England.

5 Reforms in the treatment of mentally ill people were instituted in the United States in the eighteenth century under the direction of:
   a Martha Mitchell.   c Dorothy Lynde Dix.
   b Benjamin Franklin.   d Thomas Kirkbride.

6 The "father of American psychiatry" was:
   a Sigmund Freud.   c Benjamin Rush.
   b William Menninger.   d Horace Mann.

7 The *first* treatment modalities called tranquilizers were:
   a Restraining devices.   c Sulphur baths.
   b Seclusion rooms.   d Psychotropic medications.

8 The syndrome of institutionalization refers to which one of the following?
   a Hospitalizing individuals against their will.
   b Maintaining individuals in hospitals until they are ready for discharge.
   c Promoting adaptation to hospitalization to the extent that individuals resist discharge.
   d Keeping individuals in institutions past the time when treatment is indicated.

9 Clifford Beers and his book *A Mind That Found Itself* impacted on the care of mentally ill people by:
   a Revealing the psychodynamics of mental illness.
   b Supporting the formation of community mental health centers.
   c Demonstrating a need for psychotropic drugs in the care of psychotic persons.
   d Bringing about reforms in the state hospital system of mental health care.

10 The Mental Health Act of 1946 was primarily responsible for funding the:
   a Development of community mental health centers.
   b Promotion of multidisciplinary psychiatric treatment teams.
   c Research and testing of psychotropic medications.
   d Construction of hospitals to accommodate increasing numbers of psychiatric patients.

11 In the late 1940s and early 1950s new approaches to the problem of mental illness were developed. These included *all but which one* of the following?

a Short- and long-term interventions.

b Introduction of the catchment area concept.

c Adoption of the therapeutic community concept.

d Crisis-oriented treatment programs.

12 The Omnibus Budget Reconciliation Act of 1981 provided for which one of the following?

a Curtailment in federal funding of biomedical research into the causes of mental illness.

b Increase in federal funding for purposes of early detection and prevention of mental illness.

c Maintenance of federal funding for decentralized, community-based treatment programs for mentally ill people.

d Reduction of federal funding for all mental health care services.

13 Which one of the following services is mandated at *all* community mental health centers?

a Halfway houses.

b Family therapy centers.

c Partial hospitalization.

d Suicide prevention centers.

14 Which one of the following is *not* a common practice in comprehensive community mental health centers?

a Serving the residents of a catchment area.

b Providing all clients with one-to-one therapy.

c Assisting to improve the social system in the community.

d Utilizing an interdisciplinary treatment approach.

15 Indigenous personnel working in community mental health centers usually are:

a Law-enforcement officers.

b Nonprofessional neighborhood residents.

c Psychiatric nursing consultants.

d Professional community leaders.

16 Which one of the following professions was *not* included in the core mental health disciplines?

a Psychiatric nursing.

b Clinical psychology.

c Social work.

d Activity therapy.

17 The first school of nursing in a psychiatric setting was established in the United States at:

a McLean Hospital, Massachusetts.

b Bellevue Hospital, New York.

c Boston's Psychopathic Hospital, Massachusetts.

d St. Elizabeth's Hospital, Washington, D.C.

18 Psychiatric nursing was *first* required as a part of the curriculum in all schools of nursing in:
   a 1882.   c 1934.
   b 1916.   d 1955.

19 The specialty of psychiatry was *first* given significant attention after which one of the following wars?
   a Spanish American War.   c World War II.
   b World War I.   d Korean War.

20 The psychiatrist's unique function is to:
   a Assess environmental factors. c Diagnose mental disorders.
   b Carry out physical care.   d Prescribe medications.

21 Clinical psychologists are prepared to do *all but which one* of the following activities?
   a Diagnose mental illness.
   b Treat emotionally ill persons.
   c Utilize projective techniques.
   d Administer somatic therapies to clients.

22 Which one of the following events contributed *most* to the development of the specialty of psychiatric social work?
   a Aftercare movement.   c Population explosion.
   b Introduction of milieu therapy. d World War I.

23 The role of the occupational therapist was *first* assumed by:
   a Indigenous personnel.   c Attendants.
   b Social workers.   d Nurses.

24 The concept of object relations is fundamental to the activity therapies. Implementation of this concept is primarily aimed at helping the client:
   a Express feelings, needs, and impulses.
   b Learn a new craft or hobby.
   c Practice verbal communication.
   d Explore different art forms.

25 The goals of activity therapies in a mental health setting include which one of the following?
   a To provide the client with a structured work-related program.
   b To assist in diagnostic and personality evaluations of the client.
   c To facilitate the client's return to society at large.
   d All of the above.

2 | *Psychiatric nursing and the law*

INTRODUCTION

"Psychiatric nursing is concerned with assisting individuals, families, and community groups to achieve satisfying and productive patterns of living. The law provides rules for behavioral conduct to facilitate orderly social functioning while simultaneously protecting the rights of the individual. Thus psychiatric nursing and the law affect each other greatly." * To provide optimal care for clients, nurses need to be aware of the guidelines provided by the law as care is implemented. Nurses owe it to their clients to meet their needs consistent with their rights as human beings. Nurses also owe it to themselves to be knowledgeable about the basic principles of the law as they carry out client care. The nurse as a professional person is responsible and held accountable for all nursing actions. Failure to carry out an order, administer a medication, take an appropriate action, or, on the other hand, carrying out an action, implementing an order, or administering a medication against a client's will or contrary to a client's rights may result in legal action against the nurse.

The exercises in this chapter are designed to help familiarize you with those aspects of the law which affect nursing practice.

OBJECTIVES

1. To describe methods of psychiatric admission.
2. To list examples of civil rights.
3. To categorize nursing actions in terms of the client right each one respects.

EXERCISES

1 In the space provided briefly describe what is involved in a voluntary admission.

---

*From Taylor CM: Mereness' essentials of psychiatric nursing, ed 13, St Louis, 1990, The CV Mosby Co, chap 2.

2 Mentally ill individuals frequently have a problem with insight. They do not realize that their behavior is bizarre, that they are a threat to themselves or others, or that they require professional help. In these instances involuntary admission procedures may need to be initiated by someone other than the client. There are three types of involuntary admission. In the space provided, briefly identify what is involved in each type.

a Emergency commitment

b Temporary commitment

c Extended or indefinite commitment

3 List twelve civil rights that are frequently disrupted when an individual is institutionalized. The first one has been filled in to help you get started.

a Voting _____   **g** _____
b _____   **h** _____
c _____   **i** _____
d _____   **j** _____
e _____   **k** _____
f _____   **l** _____

4 It is important that nursing care respect the rights of clients. Listed below are seven basic client rights and fifteen nursing actions involving the nurse and hospitalized clients. Categorize each action in terms of the client right it respects. Place a check in the box in the appropriate column. The first one has been filled in to help you get started.

Nursing actions	Rights of clients						
	Right to habeas corpus	Right to treatment	Right to informed consent	Right to confidentiality (privacy)	Right to independent psychiatric examination	Right to refuse treatment	Right to be free of restraints
1. Protect clients from being deprived of liberty illegally.	☑	☐	☐	☐	☐	☐	☐
2. Give clients specific and sufficient data regarding proposed nursing care.	☐	☐	☐	☐	☐	☐	☐
3. Provide clients with humane psychological and physical environment.	☐	☐	☐	☐	☐	☐	☐
4. Keep clients under constant and close supervision when they threaten self or others.	☐	☐	☐	☐	☐	☐	☐
5. Inform clients that they have the right to talk to a physician of their own choice.	☐	☐	☐	☐	☐	☐	☐
6. Instruct clients regarding the purpose, risks, and side effects of prescribed medications.	☐	☐	☐	☐	☐	☐	☐
7. Ensure clients' speedy release from illegal detension.	☐	☐	☐	☐	☐	☐	☐
8. Facilitate clients' contacts with attorneys to discuss their commitment.	☐	☐	☐	☐	☐	☐	☐
9. Develop and carry out individualized treatment plans.	☐	☐	☐	☐	☐	☐	☐
10. Withhold refused medication if it does not affect the safety of the clients or others.	☐	☐	☐	☐	☐	☐	☐
11. Tell clients of the need to share selected information regarding their condition with others involved in their care.	☐	☐	☐	☐	☐	☐	☐
12. Carry out the physician's order to medicate and seclude violent clients who are threatening others.	☐	☐	☐	☐	☐	☐	☐
13. Provide sufficient and qualified nursing staff to give clients adequate care.	☐	☐	☐	☐	☐	☐	☐
14. Review treatment plans with clients, including both their positive and negative features.	☐	☐	☐	☐	☐	☐	☐
15. Notify nursing supervisor when clients refuse treatment.	☐	☐	☐	☐	☐	☐	☐

TEST ITEMS

DIRECTIONS: Select the *best* response. (Answers appear in the Appendix.)

1 The person who is primarily responsible for assisting clients to learn about, protect, and assert their rights within the health care context is the:
  a Nursing supervisor.   c Criminal lawyer.
  b Client advocate.   d Medical doctor.

2 Which one of the following type admissions is the *least* restrictive way to obtain treatment for mental illness?
  a Emergency.   c Voluntary.
  b Indefinite.   d Extended.

3 Commitment proceedings consist of *all but which one* of the following steps?
   a Application.   b Examination.   c Detention.   d Intervention.
4 In psychiatric commitment clients usually:
   a Agree to being hospitalized.
   b Are examined by one or more physicians.
   c Are tried in a court of law.
   d Understand they are being deprived of their liberty.
5 A guardian or conservator is appointed by the court or state authorities whenever a person is:
   a Hospitalized for mental illness in a psychiatric facility.
   b Incapable of conducting his or her own affairs.
   c Found to be violent and a threat to self and others.
   d All of the above.
6 Civil rights include the right to:
   a Religious freedom.   b Education.   c Vote.   d All of the above.
7 The implementation of the Patients' Bill of Rights primarily rests with the client's:
   a Family and relatives.   b Nurse and physician.   c Lawyer.   d Judge.
8 The right to habeas corpus:
   a Establishes a human environment for the care of a hospitalized person.
   b Prohibits the disclosure of confidential material.
   c Expedites the release of a person detained illegally.
   d Arranges for a person to be examined by a physician of his or her choice.
9 Which one of the following nursing actions would be considered a violation of a client's rights?
   a Assigning the client to a small group for weekly therapy sessions.
   b Reviewing with the client the positive and negative aspects of the treatment plan.
   c Keeping the suicidal client under constant and close observation.
   d Identifying clients who are chronically ill and who will not profit from therapy.
10 One of the client's rights is the right to informed consent. For a consent to be valid it must be:
   a Given willingly and voluntarily by the client.
   b Based on adequate knowledge and information.
   c Given by a client with the legal capacity to consent.
   d All of the above.
11 Which one of the following actions taken by the nurse might result in a charge of battery being brought by the client against the nurse?
   a Physically restraining a client against his or her will.
   b Threatening to medicate a client who does not behave properly.
   c Invading the privacy of a suicidal client by keeping him or her under constant observation.
   d Interfering with a client's right to talk with an attorney.

12 A tort is *best* defined as a/an:
   a Law.   **c** Agreement.
   b Injury.   **d** Contract.

13 In a case of negligence against the nurse, the client as plaintiff must prove that:
   a A legal duty of care existed.
   b The nurse did not perform his or her duty.
   c Substantial dangers were experienced by the client.
   d All of the above.

14 The majority of lawsuits in psychiatric nursing involve which one of the following?
   a Negligence.   **c** Assault.
   b Malpractice.   **d** Battery.

15 The M'Naghten Rule used in trials involving issues of crime and sanity refers to which one of the following?
   a Test of right and wrong.   **c** Intelligence test.
   b "Irresistible impulse test."   **d** All of the above.

3

Current issues affecting the future of psychiatric nursing

INTRODUCTION

"The final years of the twentieth century will be times of challenge for psychiatric nursing. The very existence of this health care specialty is in question, while simultaneously the potential for it to make a valuable and unique contribution to the welfare of society has never been so great. Today's students of nursing will be practicing well into the twenty-first century and will be the nursing leaders of tomorrow. Since it is their nursing practice that will be affected by the way in which current issues are resolved, it is imperative that nursing students become aware of those factors which will shape the nature and scope of psychiatric nursing in the future." *

Issues are complex matters evolving from an interplay of multiple events and conditions. They are by nature controversial and raise questions that are open to discussion. As you begin the study of psychiatric nursing, it is hoped that you will not only become aware of current issues but will also be stimulated to explore the issues presented in the text as well as others you may identify and to take an active role supporting or challenging events and issues that may impact on the future of psychiatric nursing.

The exercises in this chapter are designed to help you focus on some of the current critical mental health care issues and to facilitate one role you might assume in affecting the future of psychiatric nursing.

OBJECTIVES

1. To discuss some of the effects that selected economic, social, professional, clinical, delivery system, and educational issues have on the future of psychiatric nursing and the care of mentally ill people.
2. To identify current issues affecting the future of psychiatric nursing and the care of mentally ill persons.
3. To assume an active role in supporting or challenging current issues or events that may affect the future of psychiatric nursing.

----

*From Taylor CM: Mereness' essentials of psychiatric nursing, ed 12, St Louis, 1990, The CV Mosby Co, chap 3.

EXERCISES

1 Using the following list of representative issues described in the text, discuss how they may affect the future of psychiatric nursing and the care of mentally ill people.

  a Economic issues: Inflation and economic constraints demand greater accountability from health care providers. They require the elimination of all such workers who cannot be accountable for the expenditure of their time in relation to the cost of their services.

  b Social issues: The feminist movement is a continued, organized effort of women to achieve social and economic equality with men. In spite of its positive effects, this major social trend is thought to have had at least one negative effect on the nursing profession. In an attempt to be involved in occupations with a more even distribution of men and women, fewer women are pursuing nursing as a career.

  c Professional issues: The increased move toward role blurring, in which other persons assume functions originally associated with a particular discipline, suggests that some nursing activities can be implemented at a decreased cost by less highly prepared persons.

  d Clinical issues: The long-term goals of prevention of mental illness and the promotion of mental health have been demonstrated to be the most cost-effective ways to impact on the incidence of mental illness. In spite of this fact, however, many people only support and allocate funding to short-term goals of treatment of mentally ill people because the results are more readily visible and measurable.

  e Delivery system issues: The community mental health movement is not only the most humane but also the most economical approach to the care of the emotionally ill. Unfortunately, it is doomed to failure because little effort has been made to modify treatment measures, educate health care workers, or distribute centers in a way that can best serve the greatest number of consumers.

  f Educational issues: In an attempt to view the client holistically, more and more undergraduate schools of nursing have integrated psychiatric nursing content into their curriculum. Since many nursing students are not exposed to a specific learning experience with mentally ill clients, fewer graduates from these schools are choosing psychiatric nursing as a career.

2 Refer to sources such as newspapers and magazine articles, television and radio programs, meetings and conferences, and state and national legislative action and identify current events that interest you and that you think may affect the future practice of psychiatric nursing and the care of mentally ill persons in your community. Write a letter to the appropriate party (i.e., editor of a newspaper or journal, television or radio commentator or management, conference sponsor or spokesperson, congressman, etc.) and include the following:

  a Correct name and address.

  b Article, news item, speech, legislation, etc., being addressed.

  c Date and source.

d Statement of the issue being addressed.

e Statement of agreement or disagreement with the issue.

f Rationale for the position taken.

g Your name, address, and position (i.e., student nurse).

It is suggested that you ask your instructor to check your letter before you mail it.

TEST ITEMS

DIRECTION: Select the *best* response. (Answers appear in the Appendix.)

1 Which one of the following issues is all-pervasive, directly or indirectly influencing all other issues in psychiatric nursing?

 a Clinical.   **c** Social.

 b Educational.   **d** Economic.

2 The public's increased demand for more accountability in the expenditure of time in the administration of health care is primarily associated with which one of the following issues?

 a The improved educational status of female nurses.

 b The rising incidence of mental illness.

 c The increased cost of health care services.

 d The growing concern with client's rights.

3 The use of DRGs (Diagnosis Related Groups) is expected to increase the number of mentally ill persons being cared for by:

 a Acute care facilities.   **c** Nursing homes.

 b Community agencies.   **d** Mental institutions.

4 A recent social trend that is impacting on the practice of psychiatric nursing is that:

 a Increasing numbers of women are seeking careers not traditionally associated with women.

 b More and more men are replacing women in leadership positions in nursing.

 c Fewer women are pursuing nursing careers because of the influx of men into the profession.

 d Increasing numbers of men entering nursing has favorably affected the status of all nurses.

5 The field of psychiatry has lost some of its mysteriousness with the increased:

 a Use of psychotropic agents.

 b Interest in self-help phenomenon.

 c Development of self-awareness.

 d Cost of mental health care.

6 There are about 52,000 registered nurses practicing psychiatric nursing in the United States today. According to a noted epidemiologist, by the year 2005 the need will be for about how many additional psychiatric nurses?

 a 10,000.   **c** 30,000.

 b 15,000.   **d** 55,000.

7 Some persons believe that mental illness is not really an illness but rather a reflection of societal problems. Which of the following is the *most* possible outcome of such thinking?

a Treating mentally ill persons in penal institutions.

b Returning mentally ill persons to their families.

c Removing mentally ill persons from the care of health care workers.

d Reducing the use of psychotropic drugs in the care of mentally ill persons.

8 The holistic approach to the care of mentally ill people requires that registered nurses be:

a Replaced with specially trained attendants and aides.

b Aware that their profession is jeopardized by role blurring.

c Expected to carry out traditional treatment modalities.

d Knowledgeable in both biophysical and psychosocial sciences.

9 The identity of the psychiatric nurse is *most* threatened by which one of the following?

a Holistic care.

b Self-care groups.

c Role blurring.

d Psychotropic medications.

10 The *most* cost-effective way to impact on the incidence of mental illness is to:

a Treat mentally ill persons in community mental health centers.

b Focus on the prevention of mental illness and promotion of mental health.

c Work with emotionally disturbed people in groups rather than individually.

d Concentrate on caring for acutely ill rather than chronically ill persons.

11 Which one of the following was the *initial* response among mental health care workers to the "revolving door" syndrome?

a Awareness of the enormity of the problem.

b Acceptance of the chronic nature of mental illness.

c Adoption of new and innovative treatment methods.

d Feelings of disappointment and failure.

12 The fact that it is less costly to maintain mentally ill persons outside of institutions has resulted in which one of the following *negative* effects?

a Premature discharge of mentally ill persons into the community.

b Failure to supervise the discharged person's use of psychotropic medications.

c Decreased numbers of prepared health care workers to care for discharged persons in the community.

d Increased expenditure of time and money on crisis intervention.

13 The geographical maldistribution of mental health care workers and community mental health centers has resulted in which one of the following?

 a Lack of access to adequate mental health treatment for large numbers of consumers.

 b Perpetuation of the "revolving door syndrome" in many areas.

 c Increase in the phenomenon of role blurring in community agencies.

 d Decrease in the availability of community-based self-help programs.

14 Fewer minority groups are able to complete postsecondary education programs primarily because of which one of the following?

 a Schools of higher education are closing.

 b Bilingual programs have been curtailed.

 c Costs of higher education have escalated.

 d Educational objectives are unrealistic.

15 The fact that fewer nurses are entering the specialty of psychiatric nursing is mainly attributed to the:

 a Decreasing number of persons requiring psychiatric care.

 b Integration of psychiatric content in undergraduate nursing programs.

 c Closing of institutions specific to the care of mentally ill individuals.

 d Increasing efforts to recruit nurses into other specialty areas.

Section one word games and section exercises

1 Matching: Historical perspective

DIRECTIONS: Listed below are the names of ten persons who have contributed significantly to the fields of psychiatry and psychiatric–mental health nursing. Also listed are their contributions. Match the person with the contribution by placing the number of the contribution in the space provided next to the contributor's name. The first one has been filled in to help you get started. (The solution appears in the Appendix.)

Contributions	Contributors
1. Developed a projective personality assessment test consisting of inkblots.	___ Beers
2. Known as the "father of American psychiatry."	___ Dix
3. Founded the National Committee for Mental Hygiene.	___ Freud
4. Supported a comprehensive community approach to the care of mentally ill and mentally retarded persons, emphasizing prevention as well as treatment.	___ Jarrett
	___ Kennedy
5. Presented the first course on occupational therapy.	___ Mitchell
6. Revolutionized the field of psychiatry by proposing new methods of exploring the mind.	___ Pinel
7. Liberated mentally ill persons imprisoned in chains at Bicêtre Asylum.	_1_ Rorschach
8. Represented nursing on the President's Commission on Mental Health.	___ Rush
9. Instituted reforms in the care of mentally ill persons in the United States, Canada, and Europe.	___ Tracy
10. Directed the first formal training course for psychiatric social workers.	

2 Word search

DIRECTIONS: Listed on p. 19 are 66 words hidden in the puzzle grid. They may be read up or down, forward or backward, or diagonally, but always in a straight line. Some words may overlap and some letters in the grid may be used more than once. Not all the letters in the grid will be used. Circle each word as you locate it. One word has been circled to help you get started. (The solution appears in the Appendix.)

```
N U R S I N G I N S A N E R E Z I L I U Q N A R T
O E P I D E M I O L O G Y Z E V A L U A T I O N R R
I M O S P R T S M M C I N E G O H C Y S P L Q U E
T O A E D L G S E T A C O V D A O N S F E I L E B
A T X L O R A D R U G S I N H U M A N E S X F G S
T I G O D R U Y L P P S T S P I T A H L R O I T E
L O X R M E G R E X O R C I S I N G N S Y R O D L
U N D E R W B S S D G N I R C K Y A C H U P V A P
S S E F V I A E E M U I D O C R I S I S Y I T L M
N N U S U M P F U N C C D R O R S C H T E N R M E
O D E I C O N S E N T O A B A T O Q U E G E U S T
C H I L C O N S U M E R P T N N C I T S I L O H N
L U L N O I F O R E N S I C I S B O V I O R C O E
I D I T Y O D Y S F U N C T I O N Y D A S Y L U M
N U M E A T O E V R A T D Y P O N A L C H A I S T
I X S H S S U I C M E R R T S I L A R E N E G E A
C H A I N S C K U Q E O R S Y E X O L M S G B O E
A Y T I M H O H E A L T H B C A T C H M E N T Y R
L B W A S C Y T I C I N O R H C O R O N N I D E T
A P E D O R O R S C H A C H I S I S S I N G R A I
I T M E Y A C I T A M O S M A N N O P I D G O H S
C O N S R E I C O M M U N I T Y W A I D G O A L S
O A W D I S F U N C S Y N D R O M E T O O L M I U
S A M U D E V I A N C E C H Y E X O A V E F U N E
L G N I G R U P R O F E S S I O N A L G R O U P S
```

ADDICTION	DRUGS	MANN
ADVOCATES	DYSFUNCTION	MILIEU
ALMSHOUSE	EDUCATIONAL	NURSING
ASYLUM	EMOTIONS	PINEL
BEDLAM	EPIDEMIOLOGY	PROFESSIONAL
BEERS	EVALUATION	PSYCHIATRY
BEHAVIOR	EXORCISING	PSYCHOGENIC
BELIEFS	FLOGGING	PURGING
CATCHMENT	FORENSIC	RESEARCH
CHAINS	FREUD	ROLES
CHRONICITY	GENERALIST	RORSCHACH
CLINICAL	GHEEL	RUSH
COMMUNITY	GOALS	SOCIAL
CONSENT	GROUPS	SOMATIC
CONSULTATION	HEALTH	SUICIDE
CONSUMER	HOLISTIC	SYNDROME
COPE	HOSPITAL	TEAM
COURT	HUMANITARIAN	TEMPLES
CRISIS	INHUMANE	TORT
DEVIANCE	INSANE	TRANQUILIZER
DIX	ISSUES	TREATMENT
DRGS	LAWS	TUKE

19

3 Logic problem

DIRECTIONS: Five clients—Mr. Solo, Miss Low, Mrs. Chin, Mr. Ames, and Mrs. Williams—are all inpatients in a psychiatric hospital. They are assigned to five different nurses—Mr. Mac, Ms. Cobb, Mrs. Eddy, Mr. May, and Miss Todd—who are serving as client advocates to help them with their client rights. Each nurse is working with a different client. None of the male nurses is working with a female client. Each nurse is focusing on a different client right. Using the additional clues and the grid provided below, match the clients with their nurse and the client right being served. (The solution appears in the Appendix.)

Clues:

a Mr. Solo's right to confidentiality was violated.

b Ms. Cobb's client refused medication and the nurse acknowledged the client's right to least-restrictive treatment.

c The right to habeas corpus involved one of the women clients.

d Before administering a new medication to his client, Mr. Mac gave precise information about the drug's action, side effects, and precautions to the client, acknowledging the client's right to informed consent.

e Mrs. Chin's right to treatment is observed as Miss Todd works closely with her in a nurse-client relationship.

f Mrs. Eddy is no longer working with Miss Low.

(Use an X in the boxes as you eliminate clues and an O in the boxes as you link up a clue with a client, nurse, or client right. For example, clue f indicates that Mrs. Eddy is not working with Miss Low; therefore an X has been inserted in the grid for Eddy/Low. Be sure to refer to the introductory comments in the directions for additional clues.)

Grid:		Clients					Nurses				
Client rights		Mr. Solo	Miss Low	Mrs. Chin	Mr. Ames	Mrs. Wms.	Mr. Mac	Ms. Cobb	Mrs. Eddy	Mr. May	Miss Todd
Client rights	Treatment										
	Habeas corpus										
	Confidentiality										
	Informed consent										
	Least restrictive treatment										
Nurses	Mr. Mac										
	Ms. Cobb										
	Mrs. Eddy		X								
	Mr. May										
	Miss Todd										

20

4 | *Self-awareness*

INTRODUCTION

Negative emotions such as fear, anxiety, and prejudice, as well as more positive feelings such as joy, empathy, and hope, are inextricably intertwined with beliefs that may not always be based on truth. These feelings and beliefs relate to and affect each other, sometimes clouding the nurse's perceptions of the client and interfering with the nurse's ability to focus on the client and the client's needs in an objective way.

"Whether the nurse can be a force for developing a truly therapeutic situation for the client depends on her ability to provide him with new and more positive experiences in living with other people. To accomplish this the nurse continuously strives to understand the client's behavior and the emotional needs expressed by that behavior. However, since it is the relationship between the nurse and the client that has the potential for becoming a therapeutic experience for the client, it is not sufficient for the nurse to understand only the client; in addition, she must develop self-awareness." *

Unlike self-understanding, which necessitates an in-depth self-analysis to arrive at a knowledge of why one feels and behaves as one does, self-awareness only requires that one be in touch with one's feelings, attitudes, beliefs, and actions. Through self-awareness one recognizes and acknowledges one's responses, tries to identify their source, and looks at the effect they have on one's behavior. If it is found that they interfere with relationships with others and the therapeutic care of clients, one should make an effort to modify them.

The exercises in this chapter are designed to help you to achieve greater self-awareness primarily as it applies to mental illness, psychiatric nursing, and the care of mentally ill persons.

---

*From Taylor CM: Mereness' essentials of psychiatric nursing, ed 13, St Louis, 1990, The CV Mosby Co, chap 4.

1. To differentiate between self-understanding and self-awareness.
2. To identify beliefs and feelings about psychiatric nursing, mental illness, and mentally ill persons.
3. To apply the four commonly used methods of introspection, discussion, enlarging one's experience, and role playing to the promotion of greater self-awareness.

EXERCISES

1 Differentiate between self-understanding and self-awareness.

_____

_____

_____

_____

2 Using the Johari Window as a model, identify your beliefs and feelings about psychiatric nursing, mentally ill persons, and mental illness that you have shared with others and therefore are known both to them and to you. List these in the *open window*. Also identify those feelings and beliefs that you have not shared with others and list them in the *private window*. The blind area contains beliefs and feelings of which you are unaware. They may be known to others and you may discover some of these if you are alert to verbal and nonverbal cues from others. Also, be alert to your responses to these cues. For

Open	Blind
Private	Closed

example, if you find you respond defensively, you are probably protecting yourself from developing insights in this blind area. A limited amount of space is provided for you to list new learnings in the *blind window.* The closed area is even less accessible. Decreasing the size of the blind and private areas increases the size of the open area. Achieving this goal gives you more control over your own behavior and an increased understanding of others' responses to you.

3 Inherent in developing self-awareness is a willingness to examine one's beliefs and feelings. Complete the following exercise, using the four methods of *introspection, discussion, enlarging one's experience,* and *role playing* described in the text.

    a Listed below are fifteen statements about mentally ill persons. Read each statement and, using *introspection,* reflect on your feelings and beliefs about each one. Decide whether you agree or disagree with it, then place a check in the box in the appropriate column.

Statements	Agree	Disagree
Mentally ill persons:		
1. Are hopeless and cannot be expected to change significantly.	☐	☐
2. Are different from normal people and therefore less desirable community members.	☐	☐
3. Are so fragile that they must be protected from inexperienced student nurses.	☐	☐
4. With AIDS should be isolated from mentally ill persons who are physically healthy.	☐	☐
5. Are all dangerous and need drastic treatment measures to keep them under control.	☐	☐
6. Are weak-willed individuals who could function more effectively if they tried.	☐	☐
7. Are unreliable and should not be trusted.	☐	☐
8. Have less value than healthy persons because they are not productive.	☐	☐
9. Are all aggressive and dangerous and should be locked up to protect society.	☐	☐
10. Are intellectually inferior to mentally healthy persons.	☐	☐
11. Are economically unproductive and therefore are an unaffordable luxury.	☐	☐
12. Can only be controlled by mind-altering medications.	☐	☐
13. Are defenseless and need to be protected from society.	☐	☐
14. Are too sick to be helped by student nurses.	☐	☐
15. Experience feelings that are unique and different from those of mentally healthy persons.	☐	☐

    b *Discuss* your feelings and beliefs with classmates and colleagues in a supervised classroom setting. The following questions are suggested to help focus the discussion:

       1. Can you identify the source of your feelings? (Example: a past experience; something you have read, seen, or heard).

2. What effect would communicating any of these feelings or beliefs to a mentally ill person have on your efforts to develop a nurse-client relationship?

   c Using the method of *enlarging one's experience,* seek out a client in the clinical area with whom you are unfamiliar and about whom you may have some negative perceptions. Use the tool of process recording to note both the client's behavior and your responses to the interactions.

   d In the supervised classroom setting, utilize *role playing* to enact a clinical situation with this client. It is suggested that you assume the role of the client. Follow the role playing with a group discussion.

TEST ITEMS

DIRECTIONS: Select the *best* response. (Answers appear in the Appendix.)

1 Success in creating a therapeutic situation in which positive change can occur in the client is primarily based on the nurse's ability to:

   a Develop in-depth understanding into one's behavioral patterns.
   b Alter one's behavior and attitudes toward the client.
   c Provide the client with new and positive life experiences.
   d Bring all feelings and beliefs under conscious control.

2 A nurse's primary and *most* unique tool in working therapeutically with emotionally ill clients is his or her:

   a Personality make-up.   c Emotional reactions.
   b Theoretical knowledge.   d Communication skills.

3 According to Freud, behavior is determined by beliefs and feelings that are essentially:

   a Negative.   c Pleasurable.
   b Unconscious.   d Illogical.

4 The effective practice of psychiatric nursing requires that the nurse develop self-awareness. The purpose of this effort is to accomplish which one of the following?

   a Develop an understanding of why one behaves as one does.
   b Adopt beliefs and feelings conducive to giving therapeutic care.
   c Arrive at an in-depth knowledge of one's affective responses.
   d Test and compare attitudes and beliefs with others.

5 Beliefs are thoughts that have been:

   a Proven to be true.   c Accepted as truths.
   b Found to stem from feelings. d Tested and found valid.

6 Self-awareness differs from self-understanding in that in self-awareness one:

   a Knows why one behaves and feels as one does.
   b Undergoes extensive self-examination and analysis.
   c Develops in-depth insights into one's behavior, feelings, and attitudes.
   d Explores one's behavior as a means of revealing one's beliefs and feelings.

7 Using the Johari Window as a model, the "window" that is known to one's self but is unknown to others is:

   a Private.   b Closed.   c Open.   d Blind.

8 The treatment procedure of psychoanalysis is *most* helpful in exploring which one of the following quadrants of the Johari Window?

a Private. c Open.

b Closed. d Blind.

9 In achieving self-awareness through use of the Johari Window model, enlarging the size of the open quadrant accomplishes which one of the following goals?

a Reducing the size of the closed quadrant.

b Freeing energy used to conceal beliefs and feelings from self and others.

c Achieving more control over others' responses.

d Developing insights into beliefs and thoughts concealed in the closed quadrant.

10 To increase self-awareness the nurse must be willing to do which one of the following *first?*

a Explore his or her own behavior.

b Accept the critical judgments of others.

c Relinquish defensive postures when confronted.

d Participate in meditation and/or yoga exercises.

11 Which one of the following reflective questions asked by the nurse *best* illustrates the use of *introspection?*

a "Why did the client reject me today?"

b "How does the client really feel about me?"

c "When did the client first begin to withdraw?"

d "What did I do to contribute to the client's behavior?"

12 The tool of process recording is used *most* effectively to facilitate which one of the following?

a Introspection. c Enlarging one's experience.

b Discussion. d Role playing.

13 For the process of *discussion* to be effective in promoting self-awareness, which one of the following must be present among the participants?

a Sympathy and understanding. c Enlarging one's experience.

b Spontaneity and warmth. d Respect and trust.

14 The *best* statement of a positive outcome of the process of *enlarging one's experience* is to:

a Validate one's beliefs and feelings.

b Test out one's beliefs and feelings.

c Share one's beliefs and feelings.

d Enact one's beliefs and feelings.

15 The process of *role playing* in developing self-awareness is *most* effective when it is:

a Objective. c Controversial.

b Structured. d Spontaneous.

5

Principles of psychiatric nursing

INTRODUCTION

"Being aware of one's beliefs and feelings is necessary but not sufficient for the effective practice of psychiatric nursing. To be useful, the nurse's beliefs and feelings must be organized into an internally consistent statement about the nature of human beings and their behavior. When combined with the nurse's knowledge of the scope and nature of nursing practice, these statements constitute a *philosophy* that, in turn, provides direction for developing principles of psychiatric nursing." *

Principles are rules or laws that are influenced by the prevailing beliefs about the nature of mental illness and the economic status and the cultural heritage and values of society. Seven psychiatric nursing principles have been identified and discussed in the text. They are: (1) the nurse views the client as a holistic being with a multiplicity of interrelated and interdependent needs; (2) the nurse focuses on the client's strengths and assets, not on his weaknesses and liabilities; (3) the nurse accepts the client as a unique human being who has value and worth exactly as he is; (4) the nurse has the potential for establishing a relationship with most, if not all, clients; (5) the nurse explores the client's behavior for the need it is designed to meet or the message it is communicating; (6) the nurse views the client's behavior nonjudgmentally while assisting him to learn more effective adaptations; and (7) the quality of the interaction in which the nurse engages with the client is a major determinant of the degree to which the client will be able to alter his behavioral adaptations in the direction of more satisfying, satisfactory interpersonal relationships. These seven principles of psychiatric nursing are useful in giving direction to nursing care in most, if not all, nursing situations.

The exercises in this chapter are designed to provide a practical application of selected psychiatric nursing principles to the nursing care of emotionally ill clients.

---

* From Taylor CM: Mereness' essentials of psychiatric nursing, ed 13, St Louis, 1990, The CV Mosby Co, chap 5.

1. To support nursing activities with psychiatric nursing principles.
2. To define psychiatric nursing.

EXERCISES

1 Listed below are twenty-five nursing activities and seven psychiatric nursing principles. Read each one and select the psychiatric nursing principle(s) that supports the nursing activity by placing a check in the box in the appropriate column. The first one has been filled in to help you get started.

Nursing activities	Holistic being	Strengths and assets	Unique human being	Potential for relating	Behavior communicates	Learn effective adaptations	Quality interactions
1. Encourage the client to meet those needs he is capable of meeting for himself.	☐	☑	☐	☐	☐	☐	☐
2. Listen to the client with undivided attention.	☐	☐	☐	☐	☐	☐	☐
3. Seek out the client rather than wait for the client to take the initiative.	☐	☐	☐	☐	☐	☐	☐
4. Observe the client for signs of physical illness.	☐	☐	☐	☐	☐	☐	☐
5. Help the client evaluate the consequences of his behavior.	☐	☐	☐	☐	☐	☐	☐
6. Provide the client with more positive experiences than he had experienced in the past.	☐	☐	☐	☐	☐	☐	☐
7. Treat the client with acceptance irrespective of the inappropriateness of his behavior.	☐	☐	☐	☐	☐	☐	☐
8. Recognize that emotionally ill clients are susceptible to physical as well as emotional illness.	☐	☐	☐	☐	☐	☐	☐
9. Assist the client to unlearn old, ineffective adaptations without making value judgments about them.	☐	☐	☐	☐	☐	☐	☐
10. Plan nursing care based on an understanding of the client's behavior and needs.	☐	☐	☐	☐	☐	☐	☐
11. Expose the client to a warm, caring, nurse-client relationship in which his needs take priority.	☐	☐	☐	☐	☐	☐	☐
12. Support the client's efforts to care for himself.	☐	☐	☐	☐	☐	☐	☐
13. Assess the client in relation to his social system.	☐	☐	☐	☐	☐	☐	☐
14. Give recognition and approval to the client for successful undertakings.	☐	☐	☐	☐	☐	☐	☐
15. Respect the client's right to confidentiality.	☐	☐	☐	☐	☐	☐	☐
16. Call the client by his correct surname.	☐	☐	☐	☐	☐	☐	☐
17. Establish communication with the client based on areas of similarity.	☐	☐	☐	☐	☐	☐	☐
18. Help the client to modify behavior in more productive ways.	☐	☐	☐	☐	☐	☐	☐
19. Encourage the client to make appropriate decisions when he is ready.	☐	☐	☐	☐	☐	☐	☐
20. Set limits on the client's inappropriate behaviors without being judgmental of him as a person.	☐	☐	☐	☐	☐	☐	☐
21. Help the client test out new patterns of behavior.	☐	☐	☐	☐	☐	☐	☐
22. Recognize the client's limitations simultaneous to supporting his strengths.	☐	☐	☐	☐	☐	☐	☐
23. Communicate to the client that he has the potential to change and grow.	☐	☐	☐	☐	☐	☐	☐
24. Provide an environment that supports the client's efforts to alter dysfunctional behaviors.	☐	☐	☐	☐	☐	☐	☐
25. Initiate a relationship in which genuine interest, concern, and respect are communicated to the client.	☐	☐	☐	☐	☐	☐	☐

2 Define psychiatric nursing.

_____

_____

_____

_____

DIRECTIONS: Select the *best* response. (Answers appear in the Appendix.)

1 A philosophy of nursing should reflect which of the following?
  a The nurse's feelings and beliefs.
  b An understanding of human behavior.
  c The nature of nursing practice.
  d All of the above.

2 Principles are best defined as:
  a Opinions. **b** Beliefs. **c** Rules. **d** Emotions

3 Factors influencing prevailing principles that guide the care of mentally ill persons include which of the following?
  a Economic status of society.
  b Society's beliefs about the nature of mental illness.
  c Cultural values of society.
  d All of the above.

4 The psychiatric nurse who is alert to both the physical and emotional needs of clients is working from the belief that states:
  a Each individual has some strengths and a potential for growth.
  b Human beings are complex systems of interrelated parts.
  c Each individual is unique and has inherent value.
  d All behavior is purposeful and is designed to meet a need.

5 The psychiatric nursing principle that states that the nurse focuses on the client's strengths and assets, not on his weaknesses and liabilities, is basic to which one of the following affective outcomes in the nurse?
  a Sympathy. **b** Hope. **c** Despair. **d** Impatience.

6 Which one of the following nursing activities *best* promotes autonomy in the client?
  a Encouraging the client to choose which game he wants to play.
  b Helping the client dress appropriately for visiting hours.
  c Accompanying the client to the clinic for a routine physical.
  d Sitting in conversation with the client for thirty minutes.

7 In a Judeo-Christian culture, which one of the following impressions about mentally ill clients interferes with the nurse's accepting them as valued human beings?
  a Perceiving them as being different.
  b Feeling they are unproductive.
  c Believing they are vulnerable.
  d Seeing them as needing special care.

8 Differences in feelings and behavior between mentally ill and mentally healthy persons are thought to be a matter of which of the following?

   a Deviance.   c Degree.

   b Quality.   d All of the above.

9 Use of the psychiatric nursing principle that states that the nurse has potential for establishing a relationship with most, if not all, clients is *most* facilitated by the nurse and the client sharing which of the following?

   a Emotional problems.   c Intellectual ability.

   b Experiential background.   d None of the above.

10 The nurse's willingness and ability to focus on his or her personal feelings to better understand the client's feelings is *most* specific to the development of which one of the following?

   a Communication.   c Acceptance.

   b Intimacy.   d Empathy.

11 The belief that all behavior is purposeful and designed to meet a need or to communicate a message implies that behavior is:

   a Meaningful.   c Objective.

   b Premeditated.   d Planned.

12 Which one of the following nursing activities is *best* supported by the psychiatric nursing principle that states that the nurse explores the client's behavior for the need it is designed to meet or the message it is communicating?

   a The nurse applies a knowledge of psychodynamics to clients' behavior.

   b The nurse treats clients with respect even if their behavior seems strange.

   c The nurse helps clients change ineffective behavior patterns.

   d The nurse sets limits on clients' inappropriate behavior in nonjudgmental ways.

13 All behavior observed in mentally ill persons is considered to be:

   a Dysfunctional.   c Bizarre.

   b Adaptive.   d Inappropriate.

14 Mentally ill persons are *most* vulnerable to the nurse whose care is:

   a Unskilled.   c Indifferent.

   b Inexperienced.   d Objective.

15 Psychiatric nursing may *most* correctly be described as a process through which the nurse:

   a Protects the client from life's stresses and crises.

   b Allows the client to recover at his own rate.

   c Helps the client learn the reasons for his illness.

   d Assists the client to develop a more positive self-concept.

6 _Effective communication_

INTRODUCTION

"Communication refers to the reciprocal exchange of information, ideas, beliefs, feelings, and attitudes between two persons or among a group of persons. As such it is a dynamic process requiring continual adaptations by those involved. Communication is effective when it accurately and clearly conveys the intended messages.

"The communication process is basic to all nursing practice and, when effective, greatly contributes to the development of all therapeutic relationships. Knowledge of and skill in effective communication are essential for the nurse who works with mentally ill clients because her ability to be therapeutic is highly related to the effectiveness of her communication skills." *

Mentally ill persons have been consistently exposed to ineffective patterns of communication. Incongruency and double-bind communication have been the rule rather than the exception in their interactions with people and are thought to have contributed significantly to their development of dysfunctional patterns of behavior. If mentally ill individuals are to learn more effective adaptations, they need opportunities to communicate with persons who are genuinely interested in them and who wish to help them deal with their problems. The nurse is one of the most available and appropriate members of the mental health team to render this opportunity.

In the past, communication played a relatively minor role in nursing education. Nurses' competency was measured in terms of how presentable and comfortable they made the client, how technically skilled they were in giving physical care, and how efficiently they carried out medical orders. Communication with a client was limited to seeking and giving information, to teaching very specific health-related matters, and to filling with casual conversation the awkward silences occurring in the performance of intimate physical care. Nurses who ap-

---

*From Taylor CM: Mereness' essentials of psychiatric nursing, ed 13, St Louis, 1990, The CV Mosby Co, chap 6.

proached clients, sat with them, and explored and encouraged the expression of thoughts and feelings were unique and often the target of disparagement by colleagues. Effective communication was an activity delegated to psychiatric nurses. Nurses of today who continue to function within this narrow framework are working at a distinct disadvantage to both themselves and their clients. Nursing has moved from a task-oriented to a client-centered focus. What the client thinks, believes, and feels has become increasingly important to all nurses, and, as a result, it is necessary for all nurses to acquire knowledge and skill in communicating effectively with the client and the client's family.

The exercises in this chapter are designed to help you increase your skills in identifying and utilizing effective patterns of communication.

OBJECTIVES

1. To differentiate among the four modes of communication.
2. To identify the goals of effective communication.
3. To identify and evaluate commonly used communication skills.
4. To differentiate between therapeutic and nontherapeutic nonverbal approaches.

EXERCISES

1 In the space below, briefly differentiate among the four modes of communication:

a Written communication _____

_____

_____

b Verbal communication _____

_____

_____

c Nonverbal communication _____

_____

_____

d Metacommunication _____

_____

_____

2 To be effective, the nurse's communication with the client must be guided by goals. According to the text, these goals are identified as follows: getting specific information, establishing rapport, encouraging expression of thoughts and feelings, arriving at a decision, providing reassurance, and stimulating interest. For the purposes of this exercise, two additional goals have been added: initiating a conversation and concluding a conversation. In the following exercise fifteen nursing approaches are listed. Read each one and identify which *goal or goals* guide them. The first one has been filled in to help you get started.

Nursing approaches	Goals							
	Initiating a conversation	Getting information	Establishing rapport	Encouraging expression of feelings, thoughts	Arriving at a decision	Providing reassurance	Stimulating interest	Concluding a conversation
1. "Good morning Mr. Welch. I'm Ms. Ames, a student nurse."	☑	☐	☐	☐	☐	☐	☐	☐
2. "Please tell me your name. I don't know it."	☐	☐	☐	☐	☐	☐	☐	☐
3. "I'd like to get to know you better."	☐	☐	☐	☐	☐	☐	☐	☐
4. "You might enjoy attending the music group."	☐	☐	☐	☐	☐	☐	☐	☐
5. "You seem to be having trouble deciding what to do. Let's look at your choices."	☐	☐	☐	☐	☐	☐	☐	☐
6. "It sounds like you are angry with your wife."	☐	☐	☐	☐	☐	☐	☐	☐
7. "Perhaps we can talk about this again if you like."	☐	☐	☐	☐	☐	☐	☐	☐
8. "My name is David Downs. I'll be working on this unit today."	☐	☐	☐	☐	☐	☐	☐	☐
9. "How long have you been in the hospital?"	☐	☐	☐	☐	☐	☐	☐	☐
10. "Perhaps you would find the ceramics class interesting."	☐	☐	☐	☐	☐	☐	☐	☐
11. "I see you're reading the newspaper. Is there anything interesting going on?"	☐	☐	☐	☐	☐	☐	☐	☐
12. "You seem upset today."	☐	☐	☐	☐	☐	☐	☐	☐
13. "Which dress would you like to wear?"	☐	☐	☐	☐	☐	☐	☐	☐
14. "I hope we can continue this conversation later on."	☐	☐	☐	☐	☐	☐	☐	☐
15. "I see you have combed your hair this morning."	☐	☐	☐	☐	☐	☐	☐	☐

3 One of the most misused goals in nurse-client conversations is providing reassurance. Often the nurse, keenly aware of a client's distress, low self-esteem, and negative experiences, seeks to provide immediate relief through meaningless clichés. Unfortunately, of all the conversational goals, giving reassurance is the one that does not generally lend itself to short interactions but requires a lengthy interval to be effective. Listed below are ten nursing approaches often used to provide reassurance. Read and evaluate each one in terms of its effectiveness. Place a check in the appropriate box. The first one has been filled in to help you get started.

Providing reassurance	Effective	Ineffective
1. "Don't worry."	☐	☑
2. "Let me help you think through this problem."	☐	☐
3. "I'm going to sit with you for a little while."	☐	☐
4. "Everything will be alright."	☐	☐
5. "Others are worse off than you."	☐	☐
6. "It seems you are very worried about something."	☐	☐
7. "When did you start feeling this way?"	☐	☐
8. "There is nothing to cry about."	☐	☐
9. "You shouldn't feel that way."	☐	☐
10. "Tell me about what is troubling you."	☐	☐

4 In the following situation between a nurse and a client, a variety of verbal communication skills are illustrated. Each one has been italicized and numbered. Place the number of the examples in the space provided after each communication skill. A communication skill may be illustrated more than once; an example may illustrate more than one skill. The first one has been filled in to help you get started.

Communication skills

a Clarifying _____

b Encouraging _____

c Exploring _____

d Focusing _____

e Giving information ___1___

f Introducing neutral topic _____

g Making observations _____

h Reflecting _____

i Seeking information _____

j Suggesting _____

k Understanding _____

SITUATION: A student nurse (N) approaches an elderly client (C) and initiates a conversation.

1 N   *"Good morning, Mrs. Crowe. My name is Mr. Robinson. I am your student nurse today."*

   C   "A male nurse? I didn't know there were male nurses on this floor."

2 N   *"There are two other male students besides myself assigned to this floor."* The student continues:

3 N   *"You are surprised?"*

   C   "I guess so. I'm not sure I want a man giving me care."

4 N   *"You are feeling uncomfortable about that?"*

   C   "Yes. Have you had the same preparation as the other student nurses? The women, I mean."

5 N   *"Yes. I am a senior and will be graduating at the end of the term."* Silence. Mr. Robinson observes a frown on Mrs. Crowe's face.

6 N   *"You are frowning,"* and he continues:

7 N   *"Is it my being a student or a man that troubles you?"*

   C   "Both."

8 N   *"Go on, Mrs. Crowe. Tell me what you are feeling."*

   C   "Well, now that I think about it, I guess I'm just being a silly old woman." She laughs. "A male nurse is probably as good as a female nurse." Smiling and sitting down in a chair at the bedside, Mr. Robinson says:

9 N   *"I think I am. But you're still not sure."*

   C   "I've never been taken care of by a man before. I've been very lucky. In all my 72 years I've only been in the hospital four times . . ."

10 N   *"Yes. . . ."* Mr. Robinson leans forward in his chair and maintains eye contact with Mrs. Crowe.

   C   ". . . and that was when my last four children were born."

11 N   *"Last four children?"*

12 N   He continues, *"How many children do you have?"*

   C   "Ten. Six of them were born at home. I had a terrible fear of hospitals and avoided going to them. As I said, I was very lucky. I've been healthy all my life. It's just been the last few months that I haven't felt too well. This is the first time I've been in a hospital in a very long time and I've never been cared for by a man before and. . . ." Mrs. Crowe hesitates and the student says:

13 N   *"You feel embarrassed about my giving you care?"* Mrs. Crowe nods silently then asks, "Are you going to give me a bath?"

14 N   *"Yes."*

   C   "I've been doing some of my bath for myself."

15 N   *"Fine. There is no reason to change that."* Mr. Robinson continues:

16 N   *"I'll help you with as much as you need. You will be screened and draped, and I will not expose you unnecessarily."*

   C   "And then I'll get out of bed?"

17 N   *"Yes. Perhaps you would like to sit in the solarium while I change your bed."*

   C   "That might be nice."

18 N   *"I was just out there. It's a sunny day today and nice and cheerful in the solarium with the sunshine streaming in. Did you know that there are only twenty-nine days until spring is officially here?"*

   C   "No, I didn't. I've sort of lost track of time since coming to the hospital. I used to love spring and getting out in my garden to work the soil. I always had flowers and vegetables." Mrs. Crowe pauses, then asks, "You won't forget me out in the solarium? Yesterday the nurse left me there all morning and I grew so weary."

19 N *"That must have been hard on you. It sounds like you were not able to call the nurse."*

C "No, I couldn't. There was no one to help me."

20 N *"I will leave a call bell with you in case you wish to call me."*

C "Thank you. That's a relief. . . . What did you say your name was?"

21 N *"Robinson. Tom Robinson."*

C "I'm pleased to meet you, Mr. Robinson. I think we are going to get along just fine. I'm ready for you to start my care now."

22 N *"Fine. Now as I get things ready, tell me more about yourself. You said you haven't felt too well lately. What have you been experiencing?"*

5 The text identifies several general types of nonverbal approaches, some therapeutic and some not. In the space provided in the grid below, describe two or three examples of nonverbal approaches that you consider either therapeutic or nontherapeutic. An example has been filled in to help you get started.

Nonverbal approaches	Examples	
	Therapeutic	Nontherapeutic
1. Body posture	Leaning forward	Backing away
2. Tone of voice		
3. Facial expression		

TEST ITEMS

DIRECTIONS: Select the *best* response. (Answers appear in the Appendix.)

1 Which one of the following is considered a uniquely human characteristic?

   a Language.
   b Emotions.
   c Communication.
   d Feelings.

2 More than likely, primitive man's first efforts at communication were motivated by feelings of:

    a Love.   **c** Fear.

    b Anger.   **d** Lust.

3 Man's first mode of communication was:

    a Verbal.   **c** Body language.

    b Written.   **d** Metacommunication.

4 Metacommunication *most* accurately refers to which one of the following?

    a Body language.   **c** Feedback.

    b Role expectations.   **d** Facial expressions.

5 Communication is *most* effective when verbal, nonverbal, and metacommunication are:

    a Reciprocal.   **c** Acceptable.

    b Congruent.   **d** Spontaneous.

6 Which one of the following developmental tasks must be negotiated to some degree before communication between two persons is generally effective?

    a Trust.   **c** Initiative.

    b Autonomy.   **d** Industry.

7 Which one of the following personality traits in the nurse would contribute *most* to the nurse's being able to communicate effectively with a nonverbal client?

    a Creativity.   **c** Intelligence.

    b Assertiveness.   **d** Patience.

8 In the initiation phase of the nurse-client interaction, which one of the following nursing approaches should generally be used *first*?

    a Introducing a neutral topic.

    b Focusing on the client's health.

    c Seeking factual information.

    d Introducing oneself to the client.

9 Which one of the following responses by the nurse *best* individualizes the conversation between the nurse and her client, Mr. Lowe?

    a "Tell me about yourself."   **c** "Hello, Mr. Lowe."

    b "How are you today, Mr. Lowe?" **d** "What are your hobbies?"

10 The primary reason the nurse introduces a neutral topic is to:

    a Explore a client's interests and hobbies.

    b Fill anxiety-producing silences.

    c Avoid focusing on stress-related topics.

    d Initiate a conversation with a new client.

11 Having introduced a neutral topic of conversation, nurses can *best* help their clients by doing which of the following?

    a Fill the silence by sharing their thoughts.

    b Allow their clients enough time to respond.

    c Introduce a second unrelated neutral topic.

    d None of the above.

12 The nurse will be *most* therapeutic if he or she establishes goals for each nurse-client conversation. The primary reason for this is that they help:
   a Determine the length and depth of the conversation.
   b Facilitate the evaluation of the nursing care.
   c Provide a guide to the appropriate use of approaches.
   d Communicate the nurse's genuine concern and interest.

13 Which of the following goals characterizes *most* nurse-client interactions?
   a To establish rapport.
   b To provide reassurance.
   c To get specific information.
   d All of the above.

14 Which one of the following nursing approaches is generally *least* effective in eliciting specific information from a client?
   a "What is your address?" ·
   b "Tell me your name."
   c "When did you start feeling upset with your brother?"
   d "Why do you feel so angry?"

15 The nurse and the client have been introduced and have had several brief interactions. At this time the nurse is trying to establish rapport with the client. Which one of the following approaches is *most* helpful to achieve this goal?
   a Asking the client direct questions.
   b Making observations about the client.
   c Introducing neutral topics to the client.
   d Giving the client timely advice.

16 The nurse can *most* effectively help the client to achieve the goal of arriving at a decision by doing which one of the following?
   a Giving the client advice about what is best.
   b Helping the client explore alternative choices.
   c Encouraging the client to ask a spouse what to do.
   d Sharing feelings with the client if the decision is faulty.

17 The client says to the nurse, "I'm so upset; I have so many problems and I don't know what to do." The nurse responds by asking, "Can you identify anything in particular that is upsetting you?" This is an example of:
   a Exploring.   c Clarifying.
   b Seeking information.   d Reflecting.

18 The goal of providing reassurance can be *most* effectively achieved by the nurse's saying:
   a "Everything will be alright."
   b "It seems you are very worried."
   c "There is nothing to cry about."
   d "Others are worse off than you."

19 Which one of the following nursing approaches would be *most* effective in achieving the goal of stimulating client interest?

    a "Perhaps you would enjoy going to a ceramics workshop."

    b "What would you like to do today?"

    c "You seem very thoughtful this morning."

    d "Tell me something about yourself."

20 Which one of the following goals of a nurse-client conversation usually requires a lengthy interaction?

    a Getting information.   c Providing reassurance.

    b Stimulating interest.   d Establishing rapport.

21 Basic to developing a therapeutic relationship with a mentally ill client is the nurse's having:

    a Understanding of the client's behavior.

    b Positive feelings about the client.

    c Extensive knowledge about communication skills.

    d Experience working with mentally ill persons.

22 In concluding a conversation with a client, it is *most* effective to do which one of the following?

    a Set the tone for a follow-up conversation.

    b Check that the conversation has been meaningful to the client.

    c Tell the client that you have enjoyed the conversation.

    d Promise to continue the conversation the following day.

23 A client asks the student nurse if he can go off the floor until lunchtime. Which one of the following responses by the nurse *best* illustrates double-bind communication?

    a "I don't know. You will have to ask the head nurse."

    b "I can't let you off the floor, but I'll walk you to the door."

    c "Do you think you really should leave the ward now?"

    d "We're going to play some records. Come join us."

24 The client offers to tell the nurse a secret as long as she promises not to tell anyone. Which one of the following would be the *most* appropriate response for the nurse to make?

    a "A secret? Go on, you can trust me."

    b "I'd like to hear what you have to say, but I may need to share it with the staff."

    c "I don't think you should tell me. I'll have to tell the staff."

    d "I'll listen to what you have to say, but I don't like secrets."

25 Problems in communicating with mentally ill persons arise from their having been exposed to which of the following in their past?

    a Incongruent messages.   c Double-bind communication.

    b Mistrusting relationships.   d All of the above.

7 *Nurse-client interactions*

INTRODUCTION

"Many mentally ill persons have a long history of having failed at establishing and maintaining satisfying interpersonal relationships. To the degree that the nurse's interactions with the client reflect acceptance of him and consistency in response to him, they will be therapeutic by providing experiences that are corrective of earlier, less helpful interpersonal experiences."* Of all the members of the mental health team, nurses are in the unique position of having multiple opportunities to provide these corrective experiences, showing clients that all interpersonal relationships are not to be feared and avoided.

Three different one-to-one nurse-client interactions are discussed in the text. They are differentiated on the basis of the degree of involvement and the goal of the interaction. The first type of nurse-client interaction involves a brief association, as when the nurse greets the client by name, answers a question, or sits with a client for a short conversation. In these interactions the client and nurse generally know each other, but the nurse is not primarily responsible for the client's care. The second type of nurse-client interaction is also brief. It is best characterized by the immediacy and urgency of the contact, occurring in an emergency situation. The client and nurse may or may not know each other. In this interaction the nurse is called upon to help resolve a crisis situation, such as setting limits with a client who is threatening others, intervening in a suicide attempt, sitting and listening to a client who is upset and crying, or responding to a physical emergency such as a client experiencing a hypoglycemic reaction. The third type of nurse-client interaction is the nurse-client relationship. This association is characterized by a high degree of involvement and commitment, with the nurse and client working together over an extended period of time to meet the client's physical and emotional needs. Within the framework of these nurse-client interactions, the nurse functions in a variety of overlapping and

---

*From Taylor CM: Mereness' essentials of psychiatric nursing, ed 13, St Louis, 1990, The CV Mosby Co, chap 7.

39

compatible roles as he or she attempts to meet the client's needs. These roles include the role of creator of a therapeutic milieu, socializing agent, counselor, teacher, parent surrogate, technician, and, in some instances where the nurse has advanced educational preparation, therapist.

Although the long-term nurse-client relationship is the most effective interaction for providing corrective interpersonal experiences, the role of short-term and immediate interactions should not be minimized. Within the context of any nurse-client interaction, the nurse can reach out to clients experiencing emotional pain, effectively show them that relating can be meaningful, and communicate to them a new appreciation of their worth as human beings. Factors determining the nurse's effectiveness include an understanding of human behavior, a knowledge of psychiatric nursing principles, a sensitive use of personality, an ability to comfortably assume the various roles and functions of the nurse, a thoughtful use of communication skills, an openness to reflect on his or her feelings and attitudes, and a willingness to evaluate his or her actions.

The exercises in this chapter are designed to help you gain greater understanding of nurse-client interactions and the various roles and functions of the nurse.

OBJECTIVES

1. To differentiate among three types of nurse-client interactions.
2. To list the characteristics, goals, and nursing responsibilities associated with a nurse-client relationship.
3. To plan, implement, and evaluate nursing care within the context of the nurse-client relationship.
4. To differentiate between social and therapeutic relationships.
5. To describe nursing activities associated with the different roles of the nurse.

1 Differentiate among the three types of nurse-client interactions. Read the following list of fifteen nursing actions and determine whether they are most appropriate to emergency interventions, brief nurse-client associations, or long-term nurse-client relationships. Place a check after each one in the box in the appropriate column. The first one has been filled in to help you get started.

Nursing actions	Nurse-client interactions		
	Emergency interventions	Brief associations	Long-term relationships
1. Arranges regular weekly sessions with a client.	☐	☐	☑
2. Introduces self to a client and invites him to play checkers.	☐	☐	☐
3. Waits prescribed time for client to keep appointment.	☐	☐	☐
4. Sits with new client who is crying in the dayroom.	☐	☐	☐
5. Greets a client who is known only superficially by the nurse.	☐	☐	☐
6. Reports newly admitted client's threat to escape.	☐	☐	☐
7. Responds with acceptance and consistency to testing behaviors.	☐	☐	☐
8. Intervenes in suicide attempt.	☐	☐	☐
9. Helps feed lunch to an unresponsive client.	☐	☐	☐
10. Identifies and works with client on specific problems.	☐	☐	☐
11. Prepares client for termination.	☐	☐	☐
12. Administers care to client experiencing a seizure.	☐	☐	☐
13. Helps client work through loss associated with termination.	☐	☐	☐
14. Administers routine medications to all clients on the unit.	☐	☐	☐
15. Helps client transfer positive aspects of the association to others.	☐	☐	☐

2 The nurse-client relationship usually proceeds through three developmental phases. In the grid below, list the characteristics, goals, and nursing responsibilities for the orientation, maintenance, and termination phases of the nurse-client relationship.

	Orientation	Maintenance	Termination
1. Characteristics			
2. Goals			
3. Nursing responsibilities			

3 Read the following situation involving Annie Johnson and complete the exercises as directed:

SITUATION: Annie Johnson, a 49-year-old, unmarried, obese woman, has a long history of hospitalizations for mental illness. She is usually untidy and has a strong body odor. When angry or frustrated, she tends to soil herself. Miss Johnson avoids routine shower periods by hiding from the staff. She is prone to loud, angry outbursts in which she uses gross profanity. Sometimes she brandishes chairs, wastepaper baskets, and other available articles and threatens to throw them at others.

Miss Johnson eats at every opportunity. At mealtimes she grabs food from other clients sitting at her table. Whenever she gets the chance, she rummages through the trash cans, eating any scraps of food or garbage she can find and hiding other bits of rubbish on her person or at her bedside. When not eating, looking, or begging for food, Miss Johnson sits alone in the dayroom, sleeping, rocking, or openly masturbating. Other clients tend to avoid her because of her menacing behaviors and slovenly personal habits. Miss Johnson also tends to keep away from other clients and staff, approaching them only when she wants something.

Miss Oliver, a student nurse, is assigned to Miss Johnson's unit and chooses to work with the client for the duration of her psychiatric clinical rotation. Her objective is to develop a therapeutic nurse-client relationship with Miss Johnson.

a List in a logical sequence at least four approaches that Miss Oliver might use to initiate a nurse-client relationship with Miss Johnson.

1. _____

_____

2. _____

_____

3. _____

_____

4. _____

_____

b The goal of the maintenance or working phase of the nurse-client relationship is to identify and work with the client on specific physical and emotional problems. Referring to descriptive data presented in the situation, identify and list five problems that may be the focus of the working phase of the nurse-client relationship with Miss Johnson. Be sure to include one physical problem in your list.

1. _____

_____

2. _____

_____

3. _____

_____

4. _____

_____

5. _____

_____

c Acceptance is often distorted to mean the right to feel, think, and behave without restraint. On the contrary, acceptance is not a license to behave without consideration for the rights of others. It neither condones nor approves, punishes nor condemns, but rather simply acknowledges that an individual has the right to be his own person and to respond in ways that reflect his state of being at a given time. Acceptance communicates an awareness that the person's expressions of self may not always be within the prescriptions of his society. The nurse as a professional, knowledgeable, helping, and caring person communicates the attitude and expectation that with support and guidance clients can modify their responses to function more acceptably with others without losing a basic sense of individuality.

Miss Oliver wants to communicate an attitude of acceptance to Miss Johnson. Listed below are fifteen nursing approaches that she has used with Miss Johnson at various times in their relationship. Some are accepting and therapeutic, others are nonaccepting and nontherapeutic. Evaluate each approach and place a check in the box in the appropriate column. The first one has been filled in to help you get started.

Nursing approaches	Accepting/ therapeutic	Nonaccepting/ nontherapeutic
1. "Tell me what you are feeling."	☑	☐
2. "If you don't stop misbehaving I'm going to put you in seclusion."	☐	☐
3. "Put the chair down. You may hurt someone."	☐	☐
4. "I can't let you eat other people's food. Come, have a cup of coffee with me."	☐	☐
5. "I don't like you when you behave that way."	☐	☐
6. "You are out of control. You must go into seclusion until you regain control of yourself."	☐	☐
7. "I understand you are angry with me. I would prefer you tell me this, not swear at me."	☐	☐
8. "You should tell them when you are upset."	☐	☐
9. "That's a hostile thing to say."	☐	☐
10. "Come and work with clay instead of going through the garbage."	☐	☐
11. "If you can't control yourself better, I'm going to ask the nurse to give you an injection."	☐	☐
12. "Go to your room where you can masturbate in private."	☐	☐
13. "You need to change your clothing. I will help you."	☐	☐
14. "It's OK to talk about your anger, but I can't let you hit others."	☐	☐
15. "You want to be left alone? All right. I'll come back later to see you."	☐	☐

d Consistency is an approach that has two dimensions: doing what one promises to do and doing the same thing each time. Consistency is a significant factor in the development of trust and the reduction of anxiety. By keeping promises the client learns that the nurse is someone who can be relied on to follow through on commitments and consequently is someone who can be trusted; by following a routine and responding predictably, the unexpected is taken out of a situation. It is often the unexpected that creates an element of uncertainty and contributes to the development of anxiety and insecurity, especially in emotionally ill persons. To the individual who has a dysfunctional life-style and who may be prone to or experiencing severe anxiety, the following of a predictable routine and the communication of a consistent attitude provide a degree of security that encourages more effective adaptations.

Miss Oliver collaborated with the staff to plan a consistent approach to the care of Miss Johnson. Listed below are fifteen nursing approaches that have been implemented with the client. Some are consistent and therapeutic, others are inconsistent and nontherapeutic. Evaluate each approach and place a check in the box in the appropriate column. The first one has been filled in to help you get started.

Nursing approaches	Consistent/ therapeutic	Inconsistent/ nontherapeutic
1. Spending two hours with the client every Tuesday and Friday morning.	☑	☐
2. Sitting and waiting 10-15 minutes for the client to return if she walked away.	☐	☐
3. Seeking out the client when she did not return, unless engaged with another client.	☐	☐
4. Addressing the client either as "Annie" or "Miss Johnson."	☐	☐
5. Helping the client with her hygiene on every visit.	☐	☐
6. Maintaining an accepting manner despite the client's unpredictable behavior.	☐	☐
7. Setting limits in response to the client's manipulations to prolong the visits.	☐	☐
8. Setting limits on masturbatory activities unless her embarrassment interfered.	☐	☐
9. Distracting the client with clay modeling whenever she rummaged in the garbage.	☐	☐
10. Setting limits whenever the client grabbed at other clients' food.	☐	☐
11. Bringing the client a comb and lipstick she had been promised.	☐	☐
12. Introducing the topic of termination at least once a week as the end of the relationship drew near.	☐	☐
13. Trying unsuccessfully to be accepting of the development of regressive behaviors when termination was introduced.	☐	☐
14. Avoiding a discussion of feelings of loss unless reminded to do so by the instructor.	☐	☐
15. Keeping her promise not to visit the client when the experience was over.	☐	☐

4 Listed below are ten characteristics of either *social* or *therapeutic* relationships. Differentiate between each one by placing a check in the box in the appropriate column. The first one has been filled in to help you get started.

Characteristics	Social	Therapeutic
1. The activities are goal-directed, aimed at meeting the client's needs.	☐	☑
2. The relationship develops spontaneously, without a conscious plan.	☐	☐
3. The nature of the relationship is being objectively reflected upon.	☐	☐
4. The relationship is ended in a way that encourages further relationships.	☐	☐
5. The needs of both persons involved in the relationship have equal priority.	☐	☐
6. Guidance is sought in assessing the developmental phases of the relationship.	☐	☐
7. The goal of the relationship is usually for mutual pleasure.	☐	☐
8. Activities are planned around meeting specific physical and emotional needs.	☐	☐
9. Both parties involved share mutual concern regarding reciprocal approval.	☐	☐
10. The meeting of social needs is the primary focus of the relationship.	☐	☐

5 The nurse assumes a variety of different roles within the framework of the nurse-client interactions. As the client's needs change, the nurse shifts his or her role to help make the nurse-client contacts therapeutic. In the following exercise describe nursing activities that illustrate the different roles of the nurse: technician, creator of a therapeutic milieu, socializing agent, teacher, parent surrogate, therapist, and counselor. The first one has been filled in to help you get started.

Roles of the nurse	Nursing activities
1. Technician	Carry out technical aspects of nursing care—administer medications, take vital signs, give treatments, report and record observations.
2. Creator of a therapeutic milieu	
3. Socializing agent	
4. Teacher	
5. Parent surrogate	
6. Therapist	
7. Counselor	

6 List five general nursing measures used in the administration of medications to the mentally ill:

a _____

b _____

c _____

d _____

e _____

TEST ITEMS

DIRECTIONS: Select the *best* response. (Answers appear in the Appendix.)

1 The major purpose in interacting with mentally ill clients is to:
  a Provide clients with a variety of social interactions.
  b Expose clients to experiences corrective of earlier relationships.
  c Help clients learn to trust other people again.
  d Show clients that they are unique human beings.

2 Which one of the following factors has been the *most* helpful in making clients receptive to interpersonal treatment modalities?
  a Somatic therapies.   c Psychosurgery.
  b Psychotropic drugs.   d Hospitalization.

3 Acceptance is to nonjudgmental as consistency is to:
  a Accountable.   c Subjective.
  b Discriminatory.   d Predictable.

4 A nonjudgmental attitude is reflected in a nurse who:
  a Avoids setting limits on socially unacceptable behaviors.
  b Adopts an impersonal attitude toward the client's behavior.
  c Gives approval to the client for his behavior.
  d Recognizes the client's behavior as an adaptation to stress.

5 Maintaining the same basic attitude toward the client exemplifies:
  a Acceptance.   c Consistency.
  b Objectivity.   d Understanding.

6 Nurse-client interactions can *best* be differentiated by the degree of involvement and the goals of the interaction. Which one of the following statements *best* reflects emergency intervention?
  a There need not be any previous association between the nurse and the client, and the goal resolution is immediate.
  b The nurse and the client may have some degree of involvement, and the nurse assumes a supportive role in helping others work with the client.
  c The nurse and the client know each other, and the goals of the association are long-term.
  d There is a high degree of involvement between the nurse and the client, and the goals are aimed at providing positive interpersonal experiences.

7 A client has been on the ward for 3 weeks. She rebuffs all attempts to help her relate to others. Mr. Fine, a student nurse, seeks her out daily even though he is consistently rejected. Which one of the following *best* describes the level of interaction between this client and the student?
  a Emergency intervention.
  b Orientation phase of the nurse-client relationship.
  c Maintenance phase of the nurse-client relationship.
  d Brief nurse-client association.

8 A therapeutic relationship differs from a social one in that in a *therapeutic relationship* the:

    a Needs of both parties involved must be met satisfactorily for the association to continue.

    b Goal of the association is to meet the physical and the emotional needs of both parties.

    c Nature of the association is always reflected upon in an objective way.

    d Association develops spontaneously without a conscious plan.

9 During the orientation phase of the nurse-client relationship the nurse would engage in *all but which one* of the following nursing activities?

    a Visiting the client at different times each week until a suitable meeting time is found.

    b Limiting the amount of time spent together to that which was mutually agreed upon.

    c Responding with acceptance and consistency to testing and manipulative behaviors.

    d Reflecting on feelings of frustration associated with a slow rate of progress.

10 Which one of the following client behaviors generally signals that the getting acquainted phase of the nurse-client relationship has ended?

    a Talks with the nurse.

    b Agrees to meet regularly with the nurse.

    c Decreases testing behaviors.

    d Asks about the end of the relationship.

11 The goal of the maintenance phase of the nurse-client relationship is to help clients do which one of the following?

    a Identify and resolve their problems.

    b Develop trust in the nurse.

    c See the nurse as a significant person.

    d Work through feelings of loss and despair.

12 Limit setting may be necessary when the client threatens to abuse others. If limit setting is carried out in a therapeutic manner, the client would *most* likely experience which one of the following feelings immediately?

    a Anger.   c Frustration.

    b Relief.   d Loss.

13 During the working phase of the nurse-client relationship the nurse is primarily focused on helping the client:

    a Transfer positive aspects of the relationship to others.

    b Develop insights into the cause of the client's illness.

    c Prepare for the end of the nurse-client relationship.

    d Express feelings, thoughts, and problems to the nurse.

14 In response to termination the client asks the student nurse to continue the visits after the relationship has ended. Which one of the following responses by the student would be *most* therapeutic?

a "I'd really like to visit you, but my instructor won't let me."

b "No, I can't visit. I'm afraid it wouldn't be appropriate."

c "We've had a good relationship, haven't we? It's hard to end it."

d "I don't know. Perhaps I could come visit sometime."

15 In handling their personal responses to termination, nurses need to do which one of the following?

a Delay talking about termination until their feelings of loss have subsided.

b Use the process of self-awareness to reflect on their responses to termination.

c Continue the relationship until the feelings associated with termination are resolved.

d Maintain an objective, impersonal attitude toward termination.

16 Which one of the following environmental factors would have the *most* positive effect on creating a therapeutic milieu?

a Comfortable chairs.　　　c Soothing colors.

b Accepting atmosphere.　　d Relaxing music.

17 Which one of the following clients would benefit *most* from the nurse's role of socializing agent?

a Anxious client.　　　　　c Withdrawn client.

b Depressed client.　　　　d Suicidal client.

18 The client is upset and crying uncontrollably. In her role as a counselor, a nurse can be *most* helpful by responding:

a "I can see you are very upset about something."

b "I hope you will share these feelings with your therapist."

c "You're upset now, but you will feel better tomorrow."

d "Don't cry. It can't be as bad as all that."

19 The nurse who role models for clients by dressing appropriately is utilizing which one of the following nursing roles?

a Technician.　　　　　　c Teacher.

b Therapist.　　　　　　 d Counselor.

20 Arthur Burry, an aggressive, impulsive client, needs help to control his behavior. Nurses who set limits on aggressive behavior are assuming the role of:

a Socializing agent.　　　c Therapist.

b Parent surrogate.　　　 d Counselor.

21 The nurse who administers psychotropic medications is functioning in the:

a Technical nursing role.　c Parent surrogate role.

b Therapist role.　　　　　d Counselor role.

22 The nurse collaborates with the physician in the use of psychotropic agents in the treatment of mentally ill persons. Which of the following actions would be appropriate for the nurse to take?

a Determining the most effective medication for a client.

b Suggesting an alternate route of administration.

c Obtaining a prn order of a medication.

d All of the above.

23 The ultimate goal of treatment with psychotropic medications is to:

a Maintain the client on an optimum dosage of medication for the rest of his or her life.

b Help the client function at his or her highest level with the least amount of medication.

c Assist the client to be able to monitor his or her medication plan independently.

d Help the client accept the fact that he or she will probably require medications for life.

24 Reporting and recording observations of the client's daily conversation and behavioral patterns is *most* specific to which one of the following roles of the nurse?

a Teacher.   c Technician.

b Therapist.   d Socializing agent.

25 Which of the following roles of the nurse requires advanced educational preparation?

a Teacher.   c Therapist.

b Counselor.   d All of the above.

8

The therapeutic environment

INTRODUCTION

The trend in recent years has been to treat mentally ill persons in their communities, maintaining them either in their homes or in settings with a homelike atmosphere and, at the same time, providing them with medications, group activities, and opportunities for socialization. However, community-based care is not suitable for all clients. Some persons require hospitalization. For these persons, it is equally important that the environment in which they are cared is therapeutic. "Research has documented that the environment in which the mentally ill person is treated is a major factor in enhancing or impeding the therapeutic effects of other treatment modalities. Thus, the existence of a therapeutic environment is necessary regardless of the type of setting in which a client is treated." * To be therapeutic, the environment must first recognize that clients are holistic beings and strive to meet both their physical and emotional needs. Goals of a therapeutic environment include enhancing clients' self-esteem, improving their ability to relate, and helping them become more effectively functioning members of society.

A clinical environment may be said to have two distinct, yet interrelated parts, that is, the physical environment and the socioemotional climate. The physical environment includes such elements as the size and temperature of the area and the light, sound, and furnishings in the area. The socioemotional climate, on the other hand, refers to the emotional tone set by the staff, the nature of interpersonal relationships among clients and between staff and clients, the degree of limit setting, and the effective manipulation of the physical environment to promote security and relatedness among the residents.

The nurse assumes a major role in influencing the therapeutic potential of both the physical environment and socioemotional climate. Although nurses do not generally paint walls, they can be influential in color selection. Similarly, the

---

*From Taylor CM: Mereness' essentials of psychiatric nursing, ed 13, St Louis, 1990, The CV Mosby Co, chap 8.

51

nurse can do much to enhance the physical environment by skillfully managing the light, temperature, and ventilation of the unit and by making available music, art, games, reading materials, calendars, clocks, and bulletin boards for the use of the clients. However, the nurse's greatest impact is undoubtably on the socioemotional climate. A nurse who is sensitive, caring, and responsive to the needs of clients sets a tone for a therapeutic emotional climate and serves as a role model for other staff members. Rules and regulations also influence the socioemotional climate. It is important that rules give sufficient structure to provide a sense of security without rigidity and inflexibility that might interfere with opportunities for decision making. Staff need to be aware that many clients' dysfunctional behaviors interfere with relatedness, and they should be available to interact with clients and promote socialization. Watching television, for example, can be a very effective way for clients to withdraw and avoid relating and, to that extent, may be seen as an element in the physical environment that has a negative effect on the socioemotional climate. However, a staff-led group discussion following a television viewing can promote interaction and relatedness. Encouraging clients to listen to music together; moving chairs lined up in rows into position for face-to-face interactions; promoting group rather than solitary games; and referring to clocks, calendars, and newspapers when orienting clients are all ways that nurses and other members of the staff can effectively manipulate the physical environment to enhance the socioemotional climate.

The challenge to nurses and other health care workers in psychiatric inpatient settings is to promote the therapeutic potential of the environment for those persons requiring hospitalization. The exercises in this chapter are designed to help you to focus on the hospital environment and to recognize the importance of both the physical environment and the socioemotional climate in providing a therapeutic setting where both the physical and emotional needs of mentally ill persons can be met.

OBJECTIVES

1. To differentiate between therapeutic and nontherapeutic factors that characterize the physical environment and the socioemotional climate of a psychiatric hospital setting.
2. To assess and discuss the socioemotional climate of a clinical unit.
3. To manipulate elements in the physical environment in a way that enhances the therapeutic potential of the socioemotional climate.
4. To list the major goals of a therapeutic community.

1 Listed below are twenty examples of elements characteristic of the physical environment and the socioemotional climate. Evaluate each one in terms of its being therapeutic or nontherapeutic. The first one has been filled in to help you get started.

Environmental elements	Physical environment		Socioemotional climate	
	Therapeutic	Nontherapeutic	Therapeutic	Nontherapeutic
1. Long drab corridors.	☐	☑	☐	☐
2. Two to three beds per client bedroom.	☐	☐	☐	☐
3. Nurse sitting in conversation with a client.	☐	☐	☐	☐
4. Clients eating lunch in the dining room, twenty clients per table.	☐	☐	☐	☐
5. Toilet stalls equipped with doors.	☐	☐	☐	☐
6. Week's schedule of activities tacked on the bulletin board.	☐	☐	☐	☐
7. Staff and clients avoiding an untidy, foul-smelling client.	☐	☐	☐	☐
8. Broken-down ping-pong table standing in corner of dayroom.	☐	☐	☐	☐
9. Student nurses and clients engaged in sing-along around the piano.	☐	☐	☐	☐
10. Pictureless walls.	☐	☐	☐	☐
11. Washer and dryer available for client use.	☐	☐	☐	☐
12. Attendant conducting bingo game with client group.	☐	☐	☐	☐
13. Clients wearing clean, blue hospital clothing.	☐	☐	☐	☐
14. Housekeeper locking clients in day room while corridors are mopped.	☐	☐	☐	☐
15. Student nurse orienting newly admitted client.	☐	☐	☐	☐
16. Clients sitting in dayroom, staring into space, unresponsive to each other.	☐	☐	☐	☐
17. Nonfunctioning clock and outdated calendar on dayroom wall.	☐	☐	☐	☐
18. Staff welcoming new student nurses to hospital unit.	☐	☐	☐	☐
19. Client rooms neat and spartan, devoid of personal belongings.	☐	☐	☐	☐
20. Staff member giving client cigarette moments after nurse reminded him he was on smoking restrictions.	☐	☐	☐	☐

2 Using the ten categories (or subscales from the Ward Atmosphere Scale*) listed below describe your perception of the socioemotional climate on the unit to which you are currently assigned for your clinical experience. Share this descriptive data with your classmates in a supervised classroom setting. How does the "real" compare with the "ideal"? What changes would you institute to help make the socioemotional climate of the unit you have described more therapeutic?

a Involvement _____

_____

_____

b Support _____

_____

_____

c Spontaneity _____

_____

_____

d Autonomy _____

_____

_____

e Practical orientation _____

_____

_____

f Personal problem orientation _____

_____

_____

g Anger and aggression _____

_____

_____

h Order and organization _____

_____

_____

i Program clarity _____

_____

_____

j Staff control _____

_____

_____

*See Taylor CM: Mereness' essentials of psychiatric nursing, ed 13, St Louis, 1990, The CV Mosby Co, chap 8, for a discussion of the Ward Atmosphere Scale.

3 Study the following layout of the "dayroom," focusing on the physical elements in the environment. Then in the space below describe how six physical elements could be utilized to enhance the socioemotional climate.

1. _____
   _____
2. _____
   _____
3. _____
   _____
4. _____
   _____
5. _____
   _____
6. _____
   _____

4 List at least five major goals of a therapeutic community.

1. _____
2. _____
3. _____
4. _____
5. _____

DIRECTIONS: Select the *best* response. (Answers appear in the Appendix.)

1 Historically, which one of the following factors was *most* influential in terminating the moral-treatment approach to psychiatric care?
   a Increased numbers of immigrants to the United States following the Civil War.
   b Decreased public concern with morality after the Victorian era.
   c Economic decline during the Depression in the United States.
   d Readjustment problems experienced by U.S. servicemen after World War II.

2 Dr. Maxwell Jones' book entitled *Social Psychiatry* emphasized which one of the following treatment modalities?
   a Psychotropic medications.   c Custodial care.
   b Individual psychotherapy.   d Group living.

3 A therapeutic environment is characterized as one that:
   a Focuses exclusively on clients' socioemotional needs.
   b Requires that clients participate in decision making.
   c Provides clients with a test ground for new behaviors.
   d All of the above.

4 In a therapeutic environment, rules of conduct are *most* effective if they are:
   a Implemented by the staff.
   b Established by the clients and staff.
   c Equally beneficial to all persons on the ward.
   d Consistently and strictly enforced.

5 Which of the following examples of limit setting is the *least* appropriate?
   a Expecting all clients to attend their daily activity program.
   b Restricting sexual activities among all clients.
   c Requiring all clients be bathed and dressed before breakfast.
   d Restricting smoking for all clients after one client is found to have matches illegally.

6 Which of the following is conducive to a therapeutic environment?
   a Provisions for privacy.
   b Availability of planned activities.
   c Opportunities for social interaction.
   d All of the above.

7 The primary reason for encouraging clients to wear their own clothing rather than hospital garb is to:
   a Reduce the economic strain on the hospital.
   b Provide opportunities for decision making.
   c Individualize the care of clients.
   d Brighten the environment with cheerful colors.

8 A well-equipped therapeutic environment would contain laundry facilities to assist clients to assume responsibility for their personal cleanliness. This activity would *most likely* be noted on which of the following subscales of the Ward Atmosphere Scale (WAS)?

a Support.   c Involvement.

b Spontaneity.   d Autonomy.

9 Which one of the following subscales is *not* included in the WAS?

a Staff control.   c Practical orientation.

b Physical structure.   d Program clarity.

10 To *most* effectively facilitate staff-client social interactions, a therapeutic environment would provide which one of the following?

a Glassed-in nurse's station for ease of visibility.

b Arrangement of chairs in conversational groupings.

c Large dayroom that accommodates all staff and clients.

d Dining room tables that can seat 10 to 12 clients.

11 Which one of the following *fails* to reflect full utilization of elements in the physical environment to enhance the socioemotional climate?

a Stocking the ward bookcase with reading materials and games.

b Encouraging a sing-along around the ward piano.

c Referring to the clock when orienting clients to scheduled activities.

d Moving chairs in a circle for a group discussion.

12 The network of communication in a therapeutic community primarily refers to which one of the following?

a Use of therapeutic communication skills in a nurse-client relationship.

b Open channels of communication among all staff and clients on the unit.

c Respect for chain of hierarchical communication between ward staff and hospital administrators.

d Sharing of feelings and experiences at weekly community meetings.

13 The therapeutic community is an attempt to introduce democracy into the hospital environment. Which one of the following approaches taken by the staff *best* reflects this philosophy?

a Meeting clients' needs for them.

b Encouraging clients to help plan their care.

c Continuing to make important decisions for clients.

d Setting up ward policies to regulate client behavior.

14 Therapeutic community meetings are *most* effective when they are primarily used to:

a Allow clients to ventilate their complaints.

b Facilitate social interactions between clients.

c Encourage clients to participate in problem solving.

d Communicate ward policies and rules of conduct to clients.

15 The nurse needs to take an active, responsible role on units subscribing to the concept of the therapeutic community primarily because:

a Nurses are uniquely qualified to meet clients' physical and emotional needs.

b With the discarding of many rules, care needs to be more individualized.

c Clients turn more to nurses in an environment that expects their participation.

d Other staff members are usually resistive and neglect their responsibilities.

9 *The nursing process*

INTRODUCTION

"Although the terms used to describe the nursing process vary, the process is always an adaptation of the problem-solving technique and involves the phases of assessing, diagnosing, planning, implementing, and evaluating." *

In the first phase—assessment—the nurse uses observation and interview skills to collect pertinent information about the client from the client, the client's family and friends, the client's current and previous medical records, other health care workers, and relevant textbooks and journals. In addition, the nurse validates and discusses his or her perceptions with other members of the health care team. Finally, the nurse sorts and organizes the collected data according to themes. This is a precursor to the next step in the nursing process, the diagnostic phase.

In the second phase—diagnosis—the nurse synthesizes all available assessment data and makes a nursing diagnosis. The nursing diagnosis provides direction for nursing care and is a necessary preliminary step to the third phase of the nursing process, planning.

In the planning phase the nurse develops a course of nursing action. A nursing goal or objective is stated, nursing actions through which the goal will be accomplished are outlined, and the outcome criteria, a behavioral description of the anticipated results of care, are described.

The fourth and fifth phases of the nursing process are implementation and evaluation. In implementation the nurse functions in a variety of different nursing roles while using principles of psychiatric nursing to carry out the nursing actions set forth in the plan of care. Finally, in evaluation the nurse refers to the outcome criteria described in the planning phase and notes how closely the actual results of care match the anticipated results. Generally, the closer the match, the more effective the care. Also in the phase of evaluation are the steps of revision of care and self-assessment. Having critically appraised the care as either effective or

---

*From Taylor CM: Mereness' essentials of psychiatric nursing, ed 13, St Louis, 1990, The CV Mosby Co, chap 9.

ineffective, the nurse is now in a position to identify which actions taken should be continued and which should be revised. Similarly, in self-assessment the nurse reflects on feelings, beliefs, attitudes, and behaviors and, sometimes with the help of peers, supervisors, or colleagues, alters responses that appear not to have been helpful. Although identified as the final phase, the steps involved in evaluation are often carried out in varying degrees in the other four phases of the nursing process.

In conclusion, the nursing process is an essential tool used to provide a logical and sequential approach to the identification of client problems, the development of goal-directed activities, the implementation of a course of action, and the critical appraisal of the effectiveness of care. The exercises in this chapter are designed to help you apply the steps of the nursing process to the care of persons with emotional problems.

OBJECTIVES

1. To utilize phases of the nursing process: assessment, planning, nursing diagnosis, implementation, evaluation.
2. To identify roles of the nurse as reflected through nursing actions.

EXERCISES

1 The ANA Phenomena Task Force has organized human response patterns under eight human processes: activity, cognition, ecological, emotional, interpersonal, perception, physiological, and valuation. Listed below are fifteen human response patterns. Categorize each one according to the human process under which it would most likely be classified. Place a check in the box in the appropriate column. The first one has been filled in to help you get started.

	Human processes							
Human response patterns	**Activity**	**Cognition**	**Ecological**	**Emotional**	**Interpersonal**	**Perception**	**Physiological**	**Valuation**
1. Motor behavior	☑	☐	☐	☐	☐	☐	☐	☐
2. Self-care	☐	☐	☐	☐	☐	☐	☐	☐
3. Community maintenance	☐	☐	☐	☐	☐	☐	☐	☐
4. Feeling states	☐	☐	☐	☐	☐	☐	☐	☐
5. Communication processes	☐	☐	☐	☐	☐	☐	☐	☐
6. Sexuality	☐	☐	☐	☐	☐	☐	☐	☐
7. Spirituality	☐	☐	☐	☐	☐	☐	☐	☐
8. Physical integrity	☐	☐	☐	☐	☐	☐	☐	☐
9. Thought processes	☐	☐	☐	☐	☐	☐	☐	☐
10. Sleep/arousal patterns	☐	☐	☐	☐	☐	☐	☐	☐
11. Self-concept	☐	☐	☐	☐	☐	☐	☐	☐
12. Attention	☐	☐	☐	☐	☐	☐	☐	☐
13. Elimination	☐	☐	☐	☐	☐	☐	☐	☐
14. Conduct/impulse control	☐	☐	☐	☐	☐	☐	☐	☐
15. Decision making	☐	☐	☐	☐	☐	☐	☐	☐

2 Apply the phases of the nursing process to the following situation:

SITUATION: An elderly white woman was admitted to the hospital for observation after an accident in which she was struck by a car while crossing the street against the light. At the time of admission she was awake but did not know her name or the names of any family or friends. She could not recall her address, the date, or the name of the city she was in. Her speech was slurred. Her clothing was disheveled, smelling strongly of urine. Her hair was matted and sour smelling, and her body was crusted with dirt and feces. There was evidence of old bruises. Her skin was scaly and dry to the touch. Through a Medic Alert band she was wearing on her wrist, the woman's identity was determined.

The client is a 78-year-old woman named Jennie Brown. It was learned that she had a history of hypertension and had been hospitalized the previous year with a cerebrovascular accident. At the time of her discharge from the hospital she was being maintained on anticoagulant therapy. Miss Brown's previous medical records were obtained.

The history revealed that Miss Brown is a retired schoolteacher who lives alone in a single room at a boardinghouse. Her family consists of a married younger sister who lives in another city. She has not seen her sister in many years.

Miss Brown's neighbors were contacted by hospital personnel. They seemed genuinely concerned about her condition and expressed feelings of helplessness about how to assist her. They revealed that in the past 6 months she had seemed confused. They also described how she spent more and more time alone and had been leaving the boardinghouse for days at a time without telling anyone her whereabouts. On several occasions when she failed to return, the police had been notified and were instrumental in returning her home. The local police validated these reports. They also added that Miss Brown was usually found wandering in the streets, sleeping in alleys with stray dogs, and eating out of garbage cans.

a List five sources of assessment data in this situation.

1. _____
_____

2. _____
_____

3. _____
_____

4. _____
_____

5. _____
_____

b A tool used by the nurse in the assessment phase is observation. To be most effective the nurse uses four senses to take in data about the client. Listed below are ten observations made regarding Miss Brown's general condition at the time of her current admission and the senses used to gather the data. Categorize each observation in terms of the senses used to gather the data by checking the boxes in the appropriate columns. The first one has been filled in to help you get started.

	Senses			
Observations	Seeing	Hearing	Smelling	Touching
1. Elderly white woman.	☑	☐	☐	☐
2. "My name? My name? I don't remember."	☐	☐	☐	☐
3. Disheveled clothing.	☐	☐	☐	☐
4. Skin dry and scaly.	☐	☐	☐	☐
5. Odor of urine.	☐	☐	☐	☐
6. "I don't know where I live."	☐	☐	☐	☐
7. Old bruises on the body.	☐	☐	☐	☐
8. Matted and tangled hair.	☐	☐	☐	☐
9. Slurred speech.	☐	☐	☐	☐
10. Sour-smelling hair.	☐	☐	☐	☐

c A complete nursing diagnosis consists of two parts: a statement identifying the client's concerns, problems, adaptations, or responses and a phrase suggesting a probable etiological factor contributing to the problem. Signs and/ or symptoms may also be described briefly in a nursing diagnosis statement, either after the client's response or after the etiological statement. In this exercise review the assessment data and in the space below state two appropriate nursing diagnoses for Miss Brown using both the ANA and the NANDA diagnostic frameworks.*

---

*See Taylor CM: Mereness' essentials of psychiatric nursing, ed 13, St Louis 1990, Appendix D for the NANDA Approved Nursing Diagnostic Categories and Appendix E for the ANA Classification of Human Responses of Concern for Psychiatric Mental Health Nursing Practice, Draft IV-R, Sept. 20, 1988.

d In implementing care for Miss Brown the nurse used a variety of nursing actions and nursing roles. Listed below are ten nursing actions and seven nursing roles. Categorize each action in terms of the nursing roles involved in carrying it out by checking the boxes in the appropriate columns. Keep in mind that more than one role may be involved in a nursing action. The first one has been filled in to help you get started. (See Chapter 7 for a review of nursing roles.)

Nursing actions	Nursing roles						
	Technical role	Creator of therapeutic environment	Socializing agent	Teacher	Parent surrogate	Nurse therapist	Counselor
1. Promotes interaction between Miss Brown and others.	☐	☐	☑	☐	☐	☐	☐
2. Listens to Miss Brown in a positive, empathic way.	☐	☐	☐	☐	☐	☐	☐
3. Sets limits when Miss Brown tries to get out of bed alone.	☐	☐	☐	☐	☐	☐	☐
4. Administers vitamins and antihypertensive medications to Miss Brown.	☐	☐	☐	☐	☐	☐	☐
5. Encourages Miss Brown to think through her problems.	☐	☐	☐	☐	☐	☐	☐
6. Conveys realistic reassurance by staying with Miss Brown when she is upset.	☐	☐	☐	☐	☐	☐	☐
7. Records observations and care given in client's chart.	☐	☐	☐	☐	☐	☐	☐
8. Allows client to keep some personal belongings brought in by neighbors.	☐	☐	☐	☐	☐	☐	☐
9. Feeds and bathes Miss Brown when she is confused.	☐	☐	☐	☐	☐	☐	☐
10. Invites Miss Brown to join other clients in a bingo game.	☐	☐	☐	☐	☐	☐	☐

e As Miss Brown began to recuperate, the nurse was able to interview her. List in the space below four goals of an interview.

1. _____
2. _____
3. _____
4. _____

f Interviews are generally conducted to obtain specific information. They are structured, and direct questions are used more than in a therapeutic interaction. Listed below are ten approaches that might be more appropriately used in a therapeutic situation. Using the space provided, revise each one into a direct question that could be appropriately used in Miss Brown's interview. The first one has been filled in to help you get started.

Approach	Revision
1. "Where would you like to begin?"	"What do you remember about your accident?"
2. "You are frowning."	
3. "You say you have a pain?"	
4. "Tell me about your usual diet."	
5. "I understand you have a daughter."	
6. "Tell me about your sleeping patterns."	
7. "You seem upset."	
8. "I noticed you have some bruises on your arms."	
9. "I met some of your neighbors. They seem very helpful."	
10. "Have you any feelings about returning to the boardinghouse?"	

TEST ITEMS

DIRECTIONS: Select the *best* response. (Answers appear in the Appendix.)

1 The need for an organized, efficient approach to client care became *most* apparent as a result of the:

a Nursing shortage during and after World War II.

b Development of nursing specialties in the twentieth century.

c Inadequate state of nursing education prior to World War I.

d Increasing number of dependent nursing functions in the nineteenth century.

2 Which of the following resulted from the development of the nursing care plan?
   a Standardized care among nurses.
   b Increased communication between nurses.
   c Implementation of more effective nursing care.
   d All of the above.

3 Underlying the use of the nursing process are:
   a Medical diagnostic entities.   c Sound intuitive judgments.
   b Problem-solving techniques.   d All of the above.

4 The purpose of the nursing process is to do *all but which* one of the following?
   a Define the client's problem.
   b Design a way to address the problem.
   c Review the effectiveness of care given.
   d Organize physician's orders to be carried out by nurses.

5 The ANA Phenomena Task Force has organized human response patterns under eight human processes. The response pattern of *self-care* would *most* likely be classified under which one of the following human processes?
   a Cognition.   c Activity.
   b Perception.   d Valuation.

6 The human response pattern of *community maintenance* would *most* likely be classified under which one of the following human processes?
   a Interpersonal.   c Emotional.
   b Physiological.   d Ecological.

7 Assessment data are both subjective and objective. Which one of the following is an example of objective data?
   a BP 120/80, taken by the nurse.
   b "I feel terrible," stated by the client.
   c Flushed face, observed by a staff member.
   d "He said he wanted to die," shared by the psychologist.

8 In the assessment phase of the nursing process, which one of the following sources of data is generally *most* significant?
   a Client.   c Client's family.
   b Medical records.   d Relevant textbooks.

9 When the nurse is to conduct an interview for the purpose of gathering specific information, which one of the following takes priority?
   a Identifying specific goals to be accomplished in the interview.
   b Orienting the client as to the purpose of the interview.
   c Providing a comfortable setting in which to conduct the interview.
   d Discussing the client's response to his or her problem.

10 Which one of the following examples *best* illustrates a direct approach used in interviewing a client?

a "Were you a healthy child?"

b "Can you tell me about yourself?"

c "What has happened to upset you?"

d "You have a pain in your side?"

11 *All but which one* of the following objectives is appropriate to an interview between a client and a nurse?

a Determining the client's perception of the problem.

b Discovering the duration of the problem.

c Arriving at a tentative solution to the problem.

d Gathering factual information relevant to the problem.

12 The *most* effective way for the nurse to validate information gained from observations is to:

a Make the same observation more than once.

b Check out the perceptions with the client.

c Discuss data gathered with the other staff.

d Reflect on the significance of the information.

13 Which one of the following nursing activities is a direct *precursor* to the diagnostic phase of the nursing process?

a Validating information.   c Planning care.

b Observing behavior.   d Identifying themes.

14 *All but which one* of the following activities are involved in the assessment phase of the nursing process?

a Observing behavior.

b Carrying out nursing care.

c Analyzing data.

d Validating observations.

15 A nursing diagnosis should do *all but which one* of the following?

a Identify the client's response.

b State a probable etiological factor.

c Synthesize all available assessment data.

d Identify the definitive cause of the client's response.

16 Which one of the following is the *best* statement of a nursing diagnosis?

a Altered Sensory Perception: Auditory caused by deafness.

b Altered Sleep Patterns: Insomnia due to feelings of guilt.

c Altered Impulse Patterns: Suicide attempt related to feelings of despair.

d Altered Self-Esteem precipitated by developmental stressors of adolescence.

17 The planning phase of the nursing process includes statements concerning:

a Nursing diagnosis, nursing objectives, and nursing rationale.

b Nursing goals, nursing actions, and anticipated results.

c Nursing objectives, outcome criteria, and critical appraisal.

d Nursing goals, nursing rationale, and anticipated results.

18 Factors to be considered when prioritizing nursing goals include *all but which one* of the following?

   a Stability of the client.

   b Urgency of the situation.

   c Length of contact with the client.

   d Amount of time needed to achieve the goal.

19 Which one of the following is the *best* example of an outcome criteria? Within 6 weeks the client will be:

   a Discharged symptom free.

   b Experiencing an increase in self-esteem.

   c Assuming increased responsibility for his own grooming.

   d More aware of the underlying reasons for his behavior.

20 In the implementation phase of the nursing process nurses *most* specifically:

   a Observe the client for anticipated results of care.

   b Function in a variety of nursing roles.

   c Evaluate their own responses to the client.

   d Utilize thoughtful interviewing techniques.

21 When nurses sit and listen to the client in an empathic way and provide helpful, realistic reassurance, they are assuming which one of the following nursing roles?

   a Teacher.   c Counselor.

   b Socializing agent.   d Technician.

22 Nursing roles sometimes overlap. When nurses demonstrate socially acceptable behaviors to their clients, they are assuming the roles of:

   a Counselor and socializing agent.

   b Parent surrogate and teacher.

   c Technician and nurse therapist.

   d Socializing agent and teacher.

23 Although a discrete phase in the nursing process, which one of the following phases must also overlap with *all the other phases* if it is to be fully effective?

   a Assessment.   c Implementation.

   b Planning.   d Evaluation.

24 Nurses reflect on their own feelings, beliefs, attitudes, and behaviors *primarily* during:

   a Assessment.   c Implementation.

   b Planning.   d Evaluation.

25 In the evaluation phase of the nursing process which one of the following steps generally occurs *last?*

   a Reviewing assessment data and the nursing diagnosis.

   b Studying the nursing care outlined in the nursing plan.

   c Comparing anticipated outcomes of care with actual results of care.

   d Revising or continuing the plan of care as necessary.

Section two word games and section exercises

1 Matching: Historical perspective

DIRECTIONS: Listed below are the names of six persons who have contributed significantly to the fields of psychiatry and psychiatric–mental health nursing. Also listed are their contributions. Match the person with the contribution by placing the number of the contribution in the space provided by the contributor. (The solution appears in the Appendix.)

Contributions	Contributors
1. Introduced the idea that the nurse-patient relationship has therapeutic potential. 2. Emphasized the importance of self-examination for all mental health professionals. 3. Used the hospital environment therapeutically in the treatment of the mentally ill. 4. Developed, with Lipton, the Johari Window, a tool used for increasing self-awareness. 5. Revolutionized the teaching and practice of psychiatric–mental health nursing, focusing on the therapeutic one-to-one nurse-client relationship. 6. Promoted an understanding that helpful communication is therapeutic.	_____ Freud _____ Jones _____ Luft _____ Peplau _____ Render _____ Ruesch

2 Crosshatch

DIRECTIONS: Fit the 79 words listed on p. 69 into the proper boxes. The words read left to right or top to bottom, one letter per box. TOOLS has been entered to give you a starting point. (The solution appears in the Appendix.)

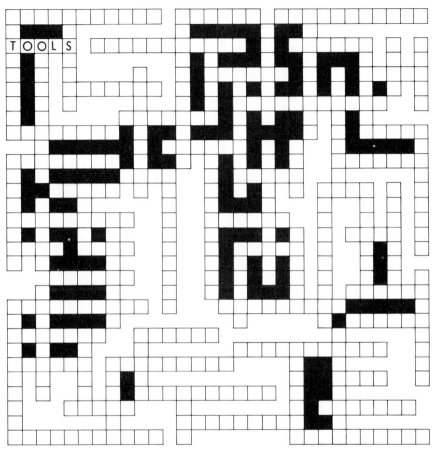

4 letters

CARE
DATA
DYAD
FEAR
GOAL
MOOD
NEED
PLAN
ROLE

5 letters

ANGER
ASSET
CHART
JONES
MORAL
NANDA
ORDER
RULES
SKILL
STAFF
TOOLS

6 letters

ACTION
ASSESS
CLICHE
CLIENT
COPING
ENERGY
JOHARI
MILIEU
NURSES
PRAISE
RELATE
SCHEMA
SORROW
STRESS
THEMES

7 letters

ANXIETY
BELIEFS
CLIMATE
EMOTION
NURTURE
PURPOSE
RESULTS
SOMATIC
TESTING

8 letters

BEHAVIOR
COMMUNAL
DURATION
DYNAMICS
ETIOLOGY
FEELINGS
FOCUSING
HOLISTIC
VALIDATE

9 letters

AWARENESS
CONGRUENT
COUNSELOR
EMERGENCY
INTERVENE
INTERVIEW
LISTENING
RATIONALE
STRENGTHS
THERAPIST

10 letters

ACCEPTANCE
ADAPTATION
DISCUSSION
EVALUATING
OBJECTIVES
REFLECTION
SUGGESTING
SYNTHESIZE

11 letters

CONSISTENCY
DISAPPROVAL
EXPLORATION
INFORMATION
INTERACTION
MAINTENANCE
SPONTANEITY
TERMINATION

3 Fill-in: Nursing interactions

DIRECTIONS: Using the definitions provided, fill in the blanks in the word list with selected content related to nursing interactions. (The solution appears in the Appendix.)

Definitions

A Rules or laws

B Disturbed interaction (two words)

C Communication goal

D Nursing role

E Therapeutic ward environment

F Implementation

G "Perhaps you'd like to take a walk."

H Parent surrogate/teacher activity (two words)

I Working phase of relationship

J Method used to increase self-awareness

K Type of nurse-client interaction

L Reporting and _____

M Nursing objective

N Results of care

O Feelings

P Major source of assessment data

Q "What other alternatives do you have?"

R Objective data

S Phase in nursing process

Word list

— — — N — — — — — — —

— — U — — — —   — — — —

R — — — — — —

— — — S — — — —

— I — — — — —

— N — — — — — — — — — —

—, — — G — — — — — — —

— — — I — —   — — — — — —

— — — N — — — — — —

— — T — — — — — — — — —

— — E — — — — — —

— — — — R — — — —

— — A —

— — — C — — — —

— — — T — — — —

— — I — — — —

— — — — O — — — —

— — — N — —

— — — — S — — — — —

4 Quote-a-crostic

DIRECTIONS: Using cues on the left, fill in the words in the list on the right. Transfer each letter in the word list to the corresponding numbered square in the puzzle grid. Shaded squares in the grid represent the end of a word. Work back and forth between grid and word list until both are completed. (Note the letters and consecutive numbers that have been entered in the grid to help in location of words.) The completed grid will be a quotation relevant to Section II of the text. The source of the quote and its author are spelled out in the boxed-in letters in the word list. One word in the list has been filled in to help you get started. (The solution appears in the Appendix.)

Cues

A Type of communication

B Conversational acknowledgment (two words)

Word list

— — ☐ — — — — — —
29 48 11 95 82 100 121 113 43

— — — — —   — — ☐
17 55 99 91 12   76 87 126

1 F		2 F	3 R	4 O	5 D		6 H	7 K		8 C	9 Q	10 O
11 A	12 B		13 K	14 F	15 L	16 D	17 B		18 K	19 N	20 E	21 C
	22 F	23 L	24 D	25 P		26 F	27 R		28 D	29 A		30 J
31 O	32 L	33 F	34 P	35 G E	36 D		37 N	38 H	39 L	40 D	41 F	
42 O		43 A	44 P	45 F	46 D		47 L	48 A		49 R	50 G A	51 I
52 P	53 H		54 D	55 B	56 N	57 P	58 F		59 L	60 J	61 I	62 D
	63 H	64 L	65 R		66 K	67 C	68 G T	69 Q	70 P		71 Q	72 J
73 H		74 R	75 M	76 B		77 D	78 K	79 J	80 E		81 O	82 A
83 J	84 H	85 M		86 K	87 B		88 D	89 C	90 P	91 B	92 I	93 O
	94 C	95 A	96 L		97 D	98 C	99 B	100 A	101 H	102 E	103 M
	104 M		105 F	106 Q	107 G T		108 D	109 C	110 O	111 F		112 C
113 A	114 I	115 D	116 F	117 O	118 N	119 G S		120 I	121 A	122 F	123 Q	124 P
	125 K	126 B	127 J	128 D	129 F		130 D	131 N	132 R	133 I	134 H	135 C

C Nursing role

__ __ __ [109] __ __ __ __ __
8 89 98 109 67 112 94 135 21

D Areas of introspection (two words)

__ __ __ __ __ __ [62] and
130 5 97 115 24 108 62

__ __ __ __ __ __ __ __ __
128 77 54 28 88 16 40 46 36

E Scot's verbal consent

__ __ [102]
20 80 102

F Technique used in the nursing process (two words)

[33] __ __ __ __ __ __
33 58 122 14 2 116 111

__ __ __ __ __ __ __
41 26 105 45 1 129 22

G Client's condition

S T A T E
119 107 50 68 [35]

H Nursing activity: instructing

___ ___ ___ ___ ___ ___ ___ [___]
6 73 63 84 53 38 101 [134]

I Socializing or psycho-
tropic _____

___ [___] ___ ___ ___
120 [92] 61 133 114

J Objective and insightful awareness of feelings of others

___ ___ ___ ___ ___ ___ [___]
79 127 30 83 51 72 [60]

K Interview questions (two words)

___ ___ ___   and   ___ ___ [___] ___
18 78 7   66 125 [13] 86

L Nurse-client relationship (three
words)

___ ___ ___ - ___ ___ - ___ [___] ___
15 64 59   47 32   23 [39] 96

M Information sought on interview

[___] ___ ___ ___
[103] 75 85 104

N End product in analysis of information

___ ___ [___] ___ ___
118 19 [131] 37 56

O Nursing action most specific to
evaluation

[___] ___ ___ ___ ___ ___ ___ ___
[81] 31 4 42 93 10 110 117

P Point of view that sees the individual as more than a mere aggregate of parts

___ ___ ___ ___ [___] ___ ___ ___
70 44 34 90 [25] 124 57 52

Q Nonverbal communication

___ [___] ___ ___ ___
71 [106] 123 69 9

R Johari _____

___ ___ [___] ___ ___ ___
49 132 [27] 65 3 74

5 6 × 6: Feelings

"Emotion turning back on itself, and not leading on to thought or action, is the element of madness."—*John Sterling**

"Fear is implanted in us as a preservative from evil; but its duty, like that of other passions, is not to overbear reason, but to assist it."—*Samuel Johnson**

Basic to existence is the experience of feelings that can be both a vitalizing and motivating force in our lives as well as an overwhelming and incapacitating influence. As caregivers we need to be sensitive to the emotions being experienced and expressed by our clients as well as be aware of our own feelings and how they are affecting our perceptions and actions. It is only with such awareness that we can hope to function effectively.

DIRECTIONS: In the following 6 × 6 grid at least twenty feelings are hidden. See how many you can locate. The letters must be connected, and a letter cannot be used more than once in a word but may be used in other words. The feeling of FEAR has been identified to help you get started. (The solution appears in the Appendix.)

A	R	L	O	O	D
N	G	E	W	M	J
U	R	E	T	A	O
A	I	L	P	H	Y
V	E	F	A	T	I
O	L	N	I	C	P

1. Fear		11.
2.		12.
3.		13.
4.		14.
5.		15.
6.		16.
7.		17.
8.		18.
9.		19.
10.		20.

*From Edwards T, editor: The new dictionary of thoughts, New York, 1954, The Standard Book Co, pp 158 and 195.

10

General systems theory and stress and adaptation
One conceptual framework

INTRODUCTION

"For nurses to practice efficiently and effectively, they must do so within the context of a conceptual framework. The purpose of a conceptual framework is to provide a logical and coherent structure through which phenomena of concern can be understood and talked about. There is no right or wrong conceptual framework. Rather, a conceptual framework is more or less appropriate; its appropriateness is determined by its applicability and utility. A conceptual framework appropriate for nursing must help explain this profession's phenomena of concern—the concepts of person, their environments, and their health as these interact between and among themselves."* The conceptual framework utilized in this text is general systems theory and the stress and adaptation theory.

General systems theory looks at the world as a complex of interrelated parts or systems. Every individual is a system unto himself, consisting of a variety of subsystems that are affected by and affecting each other. Systems may be open or closed. In a closed system the components are in relative isolation, and there is little interchange between the component parts and the environment. Human beings generally belong to open systems or relatively open systems, in which there is communication between the component parts. Figure 1 illustrates an open system, showing the interrelationships and two-way communication between the subsystems.

In a closed or relatively closed system the communication between the subsystems may be limited or nonexistent. In Figure 2 an individual maintains relatedness with several subsystems but has isolated himself from his family system.

---

*From Taylor CM: Mereness' essentials of psychiatric nursing, ed 13, St Louis, 1990, The CV Mosby Co, chap 10.

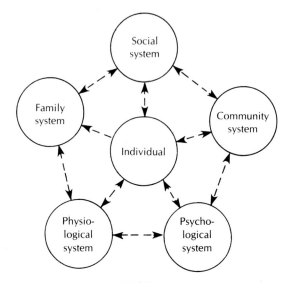

FIGURE 1

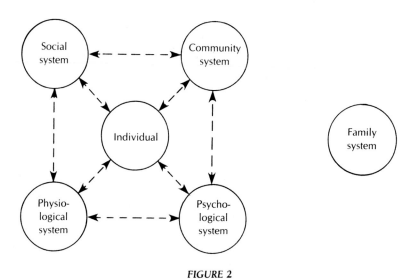

FIGURE 2

The stress and adaptation theory helps provide an understanding of the effect of stress on an individual. Stress refers to tension. Adaptation, in the general sense, refers to the individual's response, either positive or negative, to stress or tension. In its positive form it is often motivating and growth promoting; in its negative form it can be disrupting and interfere with health. Events or experiences that create stress are called stressors. They may be either developmental or situational. Developmental stressors can be anticipated. They are usually associated with challenges and tasks encountered while progressing through the stages of the life cycle. Situational stressors, on the other hand, are not predictable. They occur suddenly and unexpectedly, with little or no warning.

A knowledge of systems theory and of the theory of stress and adaptation gives nurses a conceptual framework necessary for understanding human behavior and provides them with a base for developing goals for all nursing care. The exercises in this chapter are designed to help you review several basic concepts associated with these theories as a foundation for your nursing practice.

OBJECTIVES

1. To categorize subsystems according to the system they represent.
2. To differentiate between examples of relatively open and relatively closed human systems.
3. To classify developmental and situational stressors.
4. To identify adaptations and available resources in stressful situations.

EXERCISES

1 In planning a holistic approach to client care, the nurse uses a knowledge of general systems theory that recognizes the client as being made up of multiple systems and subsystems. Listed below are five systems and fifteen examples of subsystems. Categorize each subsystem in terms of the system it represents by placing a check in the box in the appropriate column. The first one has been filled in to help you get started.

Examples of subsystems	Systems				
	Family	Social	Community	Physiological	Psychological
1. Gastrointestinal network	☐	☐	☐	☑	☐
2. Parents	☐	☐	☐	☐	☐
3. Culture	☐	☐	☐	☐	☐
4. Schools and churches	☐	☐	☐	☐	☐
5. Cardiovascular network	☐	☐	☐	☐	☐
6. Brothers and sisters	☐	☐	☐	☐	☐
7. Human needs	☐	☐	☐	☐	☐
8. Friends	☐	☐	☐	☐	☐
9. Hospitals and clinics	☐	☐	☐	☐	☐
10. Religion	☐	☐	☐	☐	☐
11. In-laws	☐	☐	☐	☐	☐
12. Feelings	☐	☐	☐	☐	☐
13. Respiratory network	☐	☐	☐	☐	☐
14. Norms and values	☐	☐	☐	☐	☐
15. Social clubs	☐	☐	☐	☐	☐

2 Although human beings generally belong to relatively open human systems, there may be instances in which they isolate themselves from their environment. At such times there is little interchange between one or more of the

subsystems. Listed below are fifteen behavioral examples of either relatively open or closed systems. Differentiate between each one by placing a check in the box in the appropriate column. The first one has been filled in to help you get started.

Behavioral examples	Relatively	
	Open system	Closed system
1. Attends local church.	☑	☐
2. Participates in civic organizations.	☐	☐
3. Ignores communications from school counselor.	☐	☐
4. Lives alone and does not socialize with others.	☐	☐
5. Volunteers to fund-raise in neighborhood.	☐	☐
6. Dies at home alone, undiscovered for 3 weeks.	☐	☐
7. Allows house to deteriorate rather than seek help.	☐	☐
8. Baby-sits with neighborhood children.	☐	☐
9. Prepares a stew for a sick relative.	☐	☐
10. Has an unlisted telephone and discourages callers.	☐	☐
11. Grooms and walks dogs at a local animal shelter.	☐	☐
12. Participates in library program to read to the elderly.	☐	☐
13. Attends and participates in PTA meetings.	☐	☐
14. Avails self of free monthly blood pressure check.	☐	☐
15. Seeks medical advice for unexplained hoarseness.	☐	☐

3 Events and experiences that create stress are called stressors. Those which can be anticipated and are predictable are developmental; those which are unexpected and unpredictable are situational. In this exercise classify each of the following events as either developmental or situational stressors by placing a check in the box in the appropriate column. The first one has been filled in to help you get started.

Events	Stressors	
	Developmental	Situational
1. Onset of diabetic symptoms.	☐	☑
2. Birth of a new baby.	☐	☐
3. Radical mastectomy.	☐	☐
4. Adolescent's rapid growth and physical changes.	☐	☐
5. Retirement from a job.	☐	☐
6. Vacation and leisure time.	☐	☐
7. Loss of possessions in a fire.	☐	☐
8. Divorce action.	☐	☐
9. Daughter marries and moves out of state.	☐	☐
10. Onset of menopausal symptoms.	☐	☐
11. Death of elderly parent.	☐	☐
12. Winning large sum of money in sweepstakes.	☐	☐
13. Adolescent son joining the army.	☐	☐
14. Promotion and raise in salary at work.	☐	☐
15. Death of spouse from chronic illness.	☐	☐

4 The following exercise consists of two parts. The first part focuses on your past responses to stressful situations; the second part looks to the future.

   a List below in the space provided, two or more events in your past that were stressful to you. Categorize each one as either a developmental or situational stressor. Briefly describe how you handled the situation, identifying any resources you may have used to help you cope.

Past events	Dev/sit	Brief description of adaptation and resources

   b List below in the space provided, two or more concerns that you are currently experiencing that are causing you stress. Identify what you are doing, or planning to do, to cope with them, including the use, or potential use, of resources.

Current concerns	Brief description of adaptation and resources

DIRECTIONS: Select the *best* response. (Answers appear in the Appendix.)

1 The first theorist to mention the role of stress as a factor in causing disease was:

   a Ludwig von Bertalanffy.   **c** Walter Cannon.

   b Kurt Lewin.   **d** Hans Selye.

2 According to general systems theory, the only true system is the:

   a Family.   **c** Individual.

   b Community.   **d** Universe.

3 The elements or components of a system are called:

   a Boundaries.   **c** Complexes.

   b Subsystems.   **d** Frameworks.

4 Kinetic energy is energy that is:

   a Currently being utilized.

   b Destroyed by input.

   c Created from matter.

   d Available for later use.

5 The process by which a system is continuously regulating itself to attain a steady state is *most* correctly known as:

   a Entropy.   **c** Wholeness.

   b Adaptation.   **d** Homeokinesis.

6 Relatively closed systems are *most* characterized by which one of the following?

   a Boundary permeability.

   b Exchange of matter with the environment.

   c Movement toward integration and growth.

   d Energy bound in maintaining a steady state.

7 Which one of the following behavioral examples *best* illustrates relatively closed human systems?

   a Baking cakes for the school bazaar.

   b Contributing to charitable organizations.

   c Living alone with three cats.

   d Acknowledging neighbors and relatives perfunctorily.

8 Positive feedback reinforces the system, thereby encouraging the maintenance of a steady state. This leads to a situation called:

   a Entrophy.   **c** Wholeness.

   b Throughput.   **d** Permeability.

9 Which one of the following examples of feedback is *least* effective?

   a Rewarding a bright student's exceptional achievements with high grades.

   b Responding to a weak student's maximum efforts with negative feedback.

   c Responding to a bright student's minimal efforts with criticism.

   d Acknowledging a weak student's maximum efforts with positive feedback.

10 A stressor may be *most* correctly defined as an event that:
    a Causes tension.
    b Promotes growth.
    c Is predictable and avoidable.
    d Gives input to the human system.

11 Which one of the following is an example of a developmental stressor?
    a Promotion at work.
    b Loss of limb in an accident.
    c Death of aging, ailing grandparent.
    d Unmarried daughter becoming pregnant.

12 Which one of the following is an example of a situational stressor?
    a Son joining army and leaving home.
    b Father retiring from work.
    c Aging grandparents dying in automobile accident.
    d Wife experiencing menopausal symptoms.

13 According to the theory of stress, a person is *most* likely to respond to a stressor in which one of the following ways?
    a Physiologically.   c Psychologically.
    b Holistically.   d Socially.

14 Problem solving in response to a stressful situation is an example of which one of the following adaptations?
    a Coping mechanisms.   c Security operations.
    b Fight-or-flight response.   d Ego defense mechanisms.

15 *All but which one* of the following statements reflect nursing goals within the framework of general systems theory and the theory of stress and adaptation?
    a To protect the human system from all stressors.
    b To increase the human system's energy potential to deal with stressors.
    c To enhance the human system's ability to adapt to stressors.
    d To decrease the potency of stressors.

11 | *Psychosocial theories of personality development*

INTRODUCTION

Personality is the reflection of the physical, emotional, cognitive, and sociocultural characteristics that uniquely combine to contribute to each person's individuality. The development of personality is a dynamic process, involving an interplay of innate biological forces, interpersonal experiences, and cultural expectations beginning at conception and continuing into maturity. "Understanding mental health and mental illness depends to a large extent on understanding the processes through which human beings develop, emotionally and cognitively. While it is imperative that the psychiatric nurse fully understand these theories, all nurses should be familiar with them, since nursing assessment and intervention for any client must be developmentally appropriate if they are to be accurate and effective."* In addition, the nurse who understands and accepts the dynamic nature of personality development will communicate the expectation that people can change and grow in a positive direction.

The exercises in this chapter are designed to help you review the characteristics of mental health as well as selected developmental theories of Sigmund Freud, Erik Erikson, Harry Stack Sullivan, and Jean Piaget.

OBJECTIVES

1. To list the personality attributes of the mentally healthy adult.
2. To identify the characteristics of the conscious, preconscious, and unconscious and the id, ego, and superego.
3. To identify the areas of the body involved with psychosexual development and the libidinal pleasures associated with each.
4. To identify the positive or negative outcomes that reflect success or failure in mastering developmental tasks.
5. To describe the interpersonal learnings that occur in each developmental era.
6. To evaluate the effect selected reflected appraisals have on the development of the self-concept.

---

*From Taylor CM: Mereness' essentials of psychiatric nursing, ed 13, St Louis, 1990, The CV Mosby Co, chap 11.

7. To identify at which stage of development selected cognitive functions are first evident.

1 List five personality attributes of the mentally healthy adult.

1.

2.

3.

4.

5.

2 Sigmund Freud's theories are referred to as intrapsychic theories because they emphasize what goes on within the individual. In the following exercises, three of his major theoretical concepts are reviewed.

a According to intrapsychic theory, there are three levels of consciousness: the conscious, preconscious or subconscious, and unconscious. These levels have been compared to an iceberg in terms of the availability of material stored within each level. As with the iceberg, the deeper the level of consciousness, the less available the content stored there. List in the space provided two characteristics of each of these three levels of consciousness. One characteristic has been filled in to help you get started.

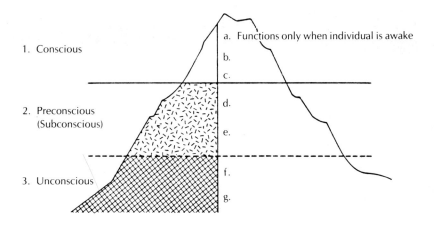

1. Conscious

2. Preconscious (Subconscious)

3. Unconscious

a. Functions only when individual is awake

b.

c.

d.

e.

f.

g.

b According to Freud there are three parts of the personality: the id, ego, and superego. It is thought that the id is innate and that the ego and superego develop subsequently as the individual comes in contact with the environment. The existence of these three parts cannot be observed directly but can be inferred through behavior. Listed below are fifteen behaviors. Identify which part of the personality is being reflected by each behavior. Place a check in the box in the appropriate column. The first one has been filled in to help you get started.

Behavior	Parts of personality		
	Id	Ego	Superego
1. Al is very self-centered, demanding, and impulsive.	☑	☐	☐
2. The infant smiles when he sees his mother approach.	☐	☐	☐
3. Joan saved her allowance to buy a new party dress.	☐	☐	☐
4. Ben feels remorse the day after drinking and behaving inappropriately.	☐	☐	☐
5. Mary had a temper tantrum when she did not get her own way.	☐	☐	☐
6. Arlene looks in the mirror and grooms herself carefully.	☐	☐	☐
7. Roy felt guilty after having lied to cover a mistake in judgment.	☐	☐	☐
8. When under stress Toni tends to overeat and drink excessively.	☐	☐	☐
9. Sue is highly motivated to succeed and studies hard at school.	☐	☐	☐
10. Tom wanted a VCR and stole one from his neighbor.	☐	☐	☐
11. The toddler tentatively touches the stove to see if it is hot.	☐	☐	☐
12. Laura feels disappointment when she fails to meet the standards she has set for herself.	☐	☐	☐
13. Jack raped Helen on their first date.	☐	☐	☐
14. Anna experienced feelings of great pleasure when she passed her biology test.	☐	☐	☐
15. The infant cried when he was wet or hungry.	☐	☐	☐

c Freud's psychosexual theory is based on the hypothesis that libidinal, or sexual, energy shifts from one part of the body to another as the individual matures physiologically. In the space provided for each stage of psychosexual personality development identify the area of the body that is invested with libidinal energy and one activity that an individual at that stage of development would consider pleasurable. An example has been filled in to help you get started.

Psychosexual stage	Area of the body	Pleasurable activities
1. Oral	Mouth	Sucking thumb (In the oral stage an infant finds thumb sucking pleasurable.)
2. Anal		
3. Phallic		
4. Latency		
5. Genital		

3 Erik Erikson's theory of personality development identifies eight ego qualities that emerge from each of the *eight ages of man*. Their emergence at a given time indicates the individual's ability to follow a social timetable for the mastery of certain basic achievements. These age-related and culturally determined achievements have become known as developmental tasks. Each task must be completed, at least in part, before the next one is achieved. Each task builds on previous ones. Difficulties mastering one task contribute to difficulties mastering subsequent ones. Mastery is affected by the nature of the relationships a person experiences as each age is negotiated. If the experiences are essentially supportive and positive, the outcomes will also tend to be positive. On the other hand, if the experiences are rejecting and negative, the result will usually be negative. These positive or negative results or outcomes are expressed behaviorally. This developmental process is a dynamic one. It was not Erikson's intent to communicate that a task once adopted was secure for all time. New experiences, positive or negative, effect changes in the outcomes.

This theory is particularly meaningful to nursing because it supports the nurse's efforts to provide clients with experiences more positive than those they had previously known. In so doing, the nurse helps clients in the mastery of developmental tasks with which they had difficulty. Success or failure negotiating Erikson's eight stages and tasks is reflected in adult verbal and nonverbal behavior. Listed below are the positive and negative outcomes for each stage and verbal responses illustrating each outcome. Match each verbal response to the outcome it best exemplifies by filling in the blanks provided. An outcome will be used only once. One outcome has been filled in to help you get started.

Positive and negative outcomes

a AUTONOMY　　　**e** GUILT　　　**i** INITIATIVE　　　**m** ROLE CONFUSION

b DESPAIR　　　**f** IDENTITY　　　**j** INTIMACY　　　**n** SHAME AND DOUBT

c EGO INTEGRITY　　　**g** INDUSTRY　　　**k** ISOLATION　　　**o** STAGNATION

d GENERATIVITY　　　**h** INFERIORITY　　　**l** MISTRUST　　　**p** TRUST

Verbal responses	Outcomes
1. "I'm such a dummy when it comes to electronics. I could never learn to use a computer."	1. _____ Inferiority _____
2. "Sure, you can borrow my lecture notes. I'll need them Friday to review for the next quiz."	2. _____
3. "I'm not certain I can. I'll ask my husband. He makes all the decisions in our house."	3. _____
4. "I just enjoy being with you—listening to you, seeing you smile, hearing you laugh. . . ."	4. _____
5. "I hate my job but I can't leave it and give up the security it provides me."	5. _____
6. "I teach art in high school and in my spare time I paint portraits."	6. _____
7. "Why do you keep asking me so many questions? What are you going to do with this information?"	7. _____
8. "I get a lot of satisfaction from doing my job thoroughly and well."	8. _____
9. "Leave me alone. I don't mean to appear rude but I am a very private person."	9. _____
10. "Thanks, I appreciate the offer. But I can do it myself."	10. _____
11. "I'm so sorry. I'll never forgive myself for not being there when you needed me."	11. _____
12. "I have emphysema and my activities are limited, but there is still a lot I can do and enjoy."	12. _____
13. "Today is the first day of the rest of my life. Where am I going? What am I going to do?"	13. _____
14. "My name is Carol. I am a nurse educator."	14. _____
15. "My husband's dead. My children don't bother with me anymore. I've got nothing to live for."	15. _____
16. "I volunteer to ask the tenants in my building to join our committee."	16. _____

4 Harry Stack Sullivan's theories are referred to as interpersonal theories, reflecting his belief that what goes on between persons is most important in personality development. In the following exercise his key concepts of interpersonal learnings and the development of the self-concept are reviewed.

a In the space provided, identify and briefly describe the interpersonal learnings that occur during each of Sullivan's developmental eras. An example has been filled in to help you get started.

Developmental era	Interpersonal learnings	Description
1. Infancy	The self-concept is learned.	The child's development of the self begins in infancy and is associated with the feeding process. If satisfaction and security are experienced during feeding, a "good-me" self-concept develops; if tension and anxiety are experienced during feeding, a "bad-me" self-concept develops.
2. Early childhood		
3. Later childhood		
4. Juvenile era		
5. Preadolescence		
6. Early adolescence		
7. Later adolescence		

b According to Sullivan, the first significant interaction occurs between the infant and his or her mothering one. This person may be male or female, may or may not be the biological parent, but is always the person who nurtures the child in the early developmental years. The mothering one communicates verbally and nonverbally to the child about his or her value and worth. These messages are called reflected appraisals and are largely responsible for the way the child first sees him- or herself. By the time the child reaches the age of 6, other persons begin to take on greater importance, gradually replacing the mothering one as the most significant figure. These persons, including other parental figures, chums, teachers, and peers, communicate additional messages about value and worth that either reinforce or revise the child's original concept of self. In developing nurse-client relationships with mentally ill individuals, the nurse has the potential for becoming a significant figure to the client. As such, the nurse can have an impact on changing the client's negative feelings of self to positive ones, based on the client's experiencing positive reflected appraisals within the framework of the therapeutic nurse-client relationship. Listed below are fifteen examples of reflected appraisals that might be observed in interactions between individuals and significant others. Categorize each appraisal in terms of the effect each might have on the development of the self-concept (good-me, bad-me, or not-me), placing a check in the box in the appropriate column. The first one has been filled in to help you get started.

Reflected appraisals	Self-concept		
	Good-me	Bad-me	Not-me
1. Follows through on promises that have been made.	☑	☐	☐
2. Insists on meeting the child's needs even after autonomy is demonstrated.	☐	☐	☐
3. Criticizes the individual unfairly.	☐	☐	☐
4. Holds the child tenderly and lovingly.	☐	☐	☐
5. Communicates extreme levels of anxiety to the child.	☐	☐	☐
6. Interferes with the individual's efforts to socialize with others.	☐	☐	☐
7. Meets the child's needs in return for the child's love.	☐	☐	☐
8. Responds with praise to the child's efforts to achieve.	☐	☐	☐
9. Respects child's individuality, opinions, and wishes.	☐	☐	☐
10. Acts unpredictably in meeting the child's needs.	☐	☐	☐
11. Ridicules the individual in front of others.	☐	☐	☐
12. Treats the individual with extreme indifference.	☐	☐	☐
13. Shares pleasure and pride in the child's growth.	☐	☐	☐
14. Ignores the child's efforts to get attention.	☐	☐	☐
15. Smiles warmly and genuinely when greeting the individual.	☐	☐	☐

c In the grid below are listed fifteen commonly observed behaviors. Each one reflects the personification of self and may be said to be the outcome of consistent exposure to significant reflected appraisals. Categorize each behavior in terms of the self-concept it reflects (good-me, bad-me, not-me), placing a check in the box in the appropriate column. The first one has been filled in to help you get started.

	Self-concept		
Behaviors	Good-me	Bad-me	Not-me
1. Expresses misgivings about one's abilities.	☐	☑	☐
2. Listens with interest to what others have to say.	☐	☐	☐
3. Responds defensively to criticism.	☐	☐	☐
4. Awakens from a terrorizing nightmare.	☐	☐	☐
5. Responds shyly when meeting new people.	☐	☐	☐
6. Dissociates all-paralyzing interpersonal anxiety.	☐	☐	☐
7. Questions consistently the reliability of others.	☐	☐	☐
8. Accepts earned praise without discomfort.	☐	☐	☐
9. Expresses trust and confidence in others.	☐	☐	☐
10. Feels comfortable with expressions of tenderness.	☐	☐	☐
11. Boasts about own accomplishments.	☐	☐	☐
12. Dissociates oneself from overwhelming experiences.	☐	☐	☐
13. Faces new challenges with anticipation.	☐	☐	☐
14. Batters spouse and children when stressed.	☐	☐	☐
15. Withdraws from reality into autistic world.	☐	☐	☐

5 Jean Piaget's theories focus on the individual's ability to think, remember, and problem solve. As with the intrapsychic, interpersonal, and cultural theories, one's cognitive functions develop sequentially and, as such, occur concurrently with the development of personality. Piaget's four stages of cognitive development are sensorimotor, preoperational, concrete operations, and formal operations. The preoperational stage is divided into two periods: preconceptual

and intuitive. Listed below are ten cognitive functions. Identify during which stage each one is *first* evident. Place a check in the box in the appropriate column. The first one has been filled in to help you get started.

Cognitive functions	Sensorimotor	Preoperational: Preconceptual	Preoperational: Intuitive	Concrete	Formal
1. Understands meaning of symbols.	☐	☑	☐	☐	☐
2. Responds to environment in an undifferentiated way.	☐	☐	☐	☐	☐
3. Engages in complex problem solving.	☐	☐	☐	☐	☐
4. Understands basic number concepts.	☐	☐	☐	☐	☐
5. Views self egocentrically.	☐	☐	☐	☐	☐
6. Masters concept of object permanence.	☐	☐	☐	☐	☐
7. Thinks abstractly.	☐	☐	☐	☐	☐
8. Thinks logically.	☐	☐	☐	☐	☐
9. Grasps concepts of past, present, and future.	☐	☐	☐	☐	☐
10. Handles more complex numerical concepts.	☐	☐	☐	☐	☐

Table header: **Stages of cognitive development**

TEST ITEMS

DIRECTIONS: Select the *best* response. (Answers appear in the Appendix.)

1 The psychosexual theory of personality development is primarily credited to which one of the following men?
  a Jean Piaget.
  b Harry Stack Sullivan.
  c Sigmund Freud.
  d Erik Erikson.

2 A pioneer in the exploration of personality development from an interpersonal theoretical framework was:
  a Abraham Maslow.
  b Harry Stack Sullivan.
  c Marie Jahoda.
  d Erik Erikson.

3 The aggregate of the physical and mental qualities of the individual as these interact in characteristic fashion with the environment is a definition of:
  a Behavior.
  b Identity.
  c Sexuality.
  d Personality.

4 Characteristics of mental health are *most* accurately described as being:
  a Culturally determined.
  b Clearly differentiated from characteristics of mental illness.
  c Relatively stable in each individual.
  d Measured as precisely as characteristics of physical health.

5 Another way of stating that emotionally mature individuals have developed the capacity for independent thinking and action is to say they have achieved:

a Self-acceptance.

b Self-determinism.

c Self-awareness.

d Self-love.

6 According to Maslow, an understanding of mental illness requires an understanding of:

a Mental health.

b Personality development.

c Human needs.

d Cognitive development.

7 The *hierarchy of human needs* recognizes which one of the following needs as taking precedence over all others?

a Safety.

b Love.

c Esteem.

d Physiologic.

8 Freud's topographical description of the psyche includes which one of the following?

a Levels of consciousness.

b Stages of development.

c Ego qualities.

d Defense mechanisms.

9 The part of the mind that only functions when the individual is awake is the:

a Unconscious.

b Conscious.

c Subconscious.

d Preconscious.

10 According to intrapsychic theory, the conscious:

a Directs rational, thoughtful responses.

b Is the storehouse for material recalled at will.

c Manifests its existence through dreams.

d Is the largest part of the mind.

11 The superego is the part of the personality that:

a Provides the source of libidinal energy.

b Operates on the basis of the pleasure principle.

c Mediates between the other parts of the personality.

d Incorporates moralistic standards of behavior.

12 According to Erikson, if the individual experiences severe inconsistency and anxiety in the stage of infancy, he will experience which one of the following behavioral outcomes?

a Mistrust.

b Shame.

c Guilt.

d Inferiority.

13 According to interpersonal theory all human behavior is directed to meeting the needs for satisfaction and security. Which one of the following reflects the need for security?

a Lust.

b Sex.

c Self-esteem.

d Elimination.

14 Piaget's theory emphasizes the role of which one of the following in cognitive development?

   a Culture.   c Fate.

   b Genetics.   d Physiology.

15 Advocates of interpersonal theory believe that dysfunctional behavior in adults results from which one of the following experiences in the early developmental years?

   a Inconsistencies and anxiety-laden relationships with the biological mother.

   b Dissociating and anxiety-generating relationships with the significant other.

   c Negative reflected appraisals communicated empathically by the significant other.

   d Failure on the part of the biological mother to consistently meet the need for satisfaction.

16 During Piaget's sensorimotor stage of cognitive development, the individual characteristically:

   a Responds in an egocentric manner.

   b Develops the tool of language.

   c Grasps numerical concepts.

   d Responds with enthusiasm to new experiences.

17 The behaviors characteristically observed during early childhood reflect a struggle for which one of the following?

   a Identity.   c Power.

   b Lust.   d Intimacy.

18 Failure to resolve the oedipal conflict satisfactorily can result in which one of the following negative behavioral outcomes?

   a Mistrust.   c Doubt.

   b Shame.   d Guilt.

19 According to interpersonal theory, during the juvenile era the child acquires the tool of:

   a Competition.   c Power.

   b Language.   d None of the above.

20 The chum relationship is *most* intense during which one of the following stages of personality development?

   a Juvenile era.   c Early adolescence.

   b Preadolescence. d Late adolescence.

21 The individual's ability to classify persons or things along more than one dimension is *first evident* during which one of the following stages of cognitive development?

   a Formal operations.   c Sensorimotor.

   b Concrete operations. d Preoperational.

22 According to Erikson, an adult's ability to develop an intimate relationship with another adult of the opposite sex is largely dependent on which one of the following?

   a Meeting a warm and caring individual.
   b Experiencing the support of significant others.
   c Feeling physical and emotional well-being.
   d Mastering previous developmental tasks satisfactorily.

23 Erikson's theory concludes that for the developmental task of generativity to be achieved the individual must do which one of the following?

   a Marry and bear children.
   b Transmit values to subsequent generations.
   c Experience satisfactory heterosexual relationships.
   d Reflect with pride on accomplishments.

24 The purpose of the life review during maturity is to:

   a Identify and master unmet developmental tasks.
   b Accept the inevitability of death.
   c Redo one's life to achieve fulfillment.
   d Reconcile the futility of old age.

25 When an individual looks forward to retirement and recalls the past with pleasure, he is experiencing which one of the following ego qualities?

   a Identity.
   b Intimacy.
   c Generativity.
   d Integrity.

12 *Anxiety*
One response to stress

Anxiety and fear are universal subjective experiences involving unpleasant tension and uneasiness. While Freud saw anxiety as occurring in response to an unknown stressor associated with an unconscious intrapsychic conflict, Sullivan viewed anxiety as the outcome of an actual or anticipated threatening interpersonal experience. Anxiety is felt in varying degrees of intensity and duration and is generally perceived as negative. Mild anxiety, although uncomfortable, is manageable and can be a stimulating and motivating force bringing about change, growth, productivity, and creativity. It can be the force that drives one to study, inspires one to produce a work of art, or moves one to seek a solution to a problem. However, as the degree of anxiety increases, effective functioning decreases.

Fear, on the other hand, occurs when an identifiable stressor threatens the existence of the system. The *fight-or-flight* response is automatically activated to provide an outlet for the physiological and psychological tension associated with fear. Since feelings of fear and anxiety cannot be readily differentiated, the fight-or-flight response is also activated when anxiety is experienced. Signs and symptoms of anxiety manifest themselves physiologically, alerting the individual to the impending threat. However, since the source of the anxiety is unknown, this automatic response is ineffective in releasing the tension, and, as a result, anxiety increases.

No one can remain in a state of anxiety indefinitely. Various adaptations are used to relieve tension and help individuals regain homeokinesis. Adaptive measures called coping mechanisms are consciously employed to help deal with stress and anxiety. Short-term coping measures, such as exercising, talking, joking and laughing, eating and drinking, chewing gum, doodling, smoking, or engaging in sexual activities give brief respite from anxiety. Long-term coping measures, such as problem solving, confront the cause of the anxiety and are generally more effective. Another adaptation to anxiety is the use of defense mechanisms, which Freud called ego defense mechanisms. They include sublimation, rationalization, isolation, regression, reaction formation, and denial and are used in conjunction with the ego defense of repression to control anxiety and to keep the conflicts contributing to the anxiety out of consciousness. Sullivan called defense mechanisms security operations. They too operate out of awareness. They are apathy, somnolent detachment, preoccupation, and selective inattention and deal with interpersonal anxiety and threats to the self-concept. Neither ego defenses nor security operations are very effective in terms of long-term adaptation because they do not encourage the individual to deal with stress and anxiety in reality-based ways.

"Because anxiety is a basic factor in the development and manifestation of human behavior, it is necessary for the nurse to acquire an in-depth understanding of its characteristics, origin, and the usual adaptations to it."* The exercises in this chapter are designed to help you to increase your understanding of anxiety, its development, and the adaptations to it.

OBJECTIVES

1. To differentiate between intrapsychic and interpersonal perceptions of anxiety.
2. To reflect on one's personal responses to stressors that contribute to the development of anxiety.
3. To differentiate among coping measures, ego defense mechanisms, and security operations.

EXERCISES

1 Listed below are ten statements about anxiety that reflect the intrapsychic theory of Sigmund Freud or the interpersonal theory of Harry Stack Sullivan. In this exercise classify each statement as intrapsychic and/or interpersonal by placing a check in the boxes in the appropriate columns. The first one has been filled in to help you get started.

Statements	Intrapsychic	Interpersonal
Anxiety is:		
1. Experienced in relationships with others.	☐	☑
2. Associated with experiences involving separation.	☐	☐
3. Manifested in responses to disapproval from significant others.	☐	☐
4. The result of unconscious conflict between id and superego.	☐	☐
5. Experienced when the need for security is not met.	☐	☐
6. Controlled by adaptive measures called ego defenses.	☐	☐
7. Communicated in an empathic manner.	☐	☐
8. The result of a threat to biological integrity.	☐	☐
9. Controlled by adaptive measures called security operations.	☐	☐
10. Threatening to the self-concept.	☐	☐

*From Taylor CM: Mereness' essentials of psychiatric nursing, ed 13, St Louis, 1990, The CV Mosby Co, chap 12.

95

2 Self-awareness

As nurses reflect on personal stressors that contribute to the development of anxiety, they develop a greater appreciation of anxiety in others and the effect stress and anxiety have on the ability of an individual to function effectively. This exercise consists of two parts, one using Freudian theory and the other using Sullivanian theory. It will help you develop increased self-awareness as it applies to an understanding of anxiety and the effect anxiety has on functioning.

a When anxiety becomes excessive, it interferes with functioning. According to Freudian theory, psychic energy is used to keep anxiety-provoking conflicts out of consciousness. As more and more energy is used by the ego to maintain repression, less energy is available for life's other activities. Listed below are five ego functions. In the space provided, reflect on your own responses to stressors in the past and describe the effect anxiety had on your functioning. For each of the identified ego functions give a personal example of normal or enhanced functioning as well as disrupted functioning when anxiety was high. An example has been filled in to help you get started. (Space is also provided so that you may enter your own example for the ego function of evaluation of reality.)

Ego functions	Normal or enhanced functioning	Disrupted functioning
1. Evaluation of reality: Differentiation of real world from fantasy or dream world, insight, judgment.	I awoke from a dream and was aware it was a dream. I reflected on it with little anxiety. – – – – – – – – – – – – –	I awoke in a panic, feeling frightened by a dream. For a moment I was confused and did not realize I had been dreaming. – – – – – – – – – – – –
2. Use of cognitive abilities: Memory, thinking, learning, comprehension.		
3. Problem solving: Identification of a problem and a reasonable solution.		
4. Control of instinctual drives: Postponement of pleasure; appropriate expression of sexual and aggressive feelings.		
5. Development of relationships with others.		

b According to Sullivan, anxiety is a distressing feeling accompanied by somatic experiences as well as emotional sensations of impending doom. Furthermore, anxiety is interpersonal, occurring as a result of one or more of the following phenomena: (1) negative reflected appraisals and feelings of disapproval from real or fantasied significant others, (2) unmet satisfaction and/or security needs, and (3) empathized anxiety. In the space provided, describe a personal experience that illustrates each of Sullivan's theoretical considerations about anxiety. An example has been filled in to help you get started. (Space is also provided so that you may enter your own examples of somatic symptoms.)

Theoretical considerations about anxiety	Personal experiences
1. Somatic symptoms: Describe any physical symptoms you experienced during an anxiety-provoking situation.	Faced with a job interview, I experienced palpitations and shortness of breath.
2. Emotional sensations: Describe any feelings you experienced during an anxiety-provoking situation.	
3. Negative reflected appraisals: Describe a situation in which you experienced disapproval from a significant person and the effect it had on you.	
4. Unmet satisfaction and/or security needs: Describe a situation in which your need for satisfaction and/or security was threatened.	
5. Empathized anxiety: Describe a situation in which you were not anxious until you picked up, or empathized, anxiety in another person.	

3 Listed below are twenty-five mental mechanisms (ego defenses, security operations, and coping measures) and twenty-five behavioral examples, one for each mechanism. Match the mental mechanisms with the behavioral examples by placing the number of each example in the space provided by the mechanism. The first one has been filled in to help you get started.

Behavioral examples	Mental mechanisms
1. Bob took out his on-the-job frustrations on his wife and children.	—— Apathy
2. Six months after the death of his son, Jeff could discuss it without experiencing earlier painful feelings.	—— Compensation
3. Linda called in sick when she failed to complete a report on time.	—— Denial
4. Following a particularly controversial union meeting, Lennie came home and went to sleep.	_1_ Displacement
5. Frank made a concerted, conscious effort to put his disappointments out of mind.	—— Drinking
6. Shirley deals with stress by consuming six martinis every night.	—— Eating
7. Joe expressed indifference when he failed to get a much sought-after job.	—— Identification
8. After losing his temper at his girlfriend, Daryl brought her flowers.	—— Isolation
9. Lynn says no to cocaine, having adopted her parents' values rejecting the use of drugs.	—— Pacing
10. Before making an important decision, Marie reflected on her alternative choices.	—— Pleading sick
11. Arthur's wife is in labor, and he works off his tension by walking the hospital corridors.	—— Preoccupation
12. Louis carries a four-leaf clover and rabbit's foot for good luck.	—— Problem solving
13. Although Dick was overly polite, always smiling and joking, his humor was sarcastic and hostile.	—— Projection
14. Luther blames his wife's frigidity for his own infidelity.	—— Rationalization
15. Chester finds that sharing his worries with his friend helps to relieve his anxiety.	—— Reaction formation
16. Helen is unable to face the reality that she has a terminal illness.	—— Regression
17. Alice's recent weight gain of 55 pounds reflects her characteristic response to stress.	—— Repression
18. Todd was deep in his own thoughts, rehearsing a speech he had to make the next day.	—— Selective inattention
19. Although usually independent, Sally becomes very clinging and helpless when physically ill.	—— Smoking
20. Maggie finds that swimming at the local spa helps her to relax.	—— Somnolent detachment
21. Two years after graduation, Joan meets a high school rival and cannot recall her name.	—— Sublimation
22. Chuck is awkward in sports activities and puts his energies into being an honor student.	—— Suppression
23. Although the TV was turned on, Sam did not hear the program because he was studying.	—— Symbolization/ condensation
24. Nathan finds writing stressful and chain-smokes when he has to prepare written reports.	—— Talking
25. Bea feels awkward socially and avoids dating by saying she prefers to sit and watch TV alone.	—— Undoing

TEST ITEMS

DIRECTIONS: Select the *best* response. (Answers appear in the Appendix.)

1 Which one of the following is *more* true of anxiety functioning as an adaptation than as a stressor?

  a Signals the system that homeokinesis is not being maintained.

  b Puts the system into a state of stress.

  c Sees anxiety as a desirable and pleasurable emotion.

  d Compounds rather than relieves the original stress.

2 The emotion of fear is *most* specifically dealt with through the use of which one of the following adaptations?

  a Ego defense mechanisms.   **c** Security operations.

  b Fight-or-flight responses.   **d** Coping measures.

3 Ego defense mechanisms are *least* pathological when:

a One or two mechanisms are used exclusively.

b A variety of mechanisms are used sparingly.

c Mechanisms effectively obscure reality.

d Mechanisms reduce anxiety and increase security.

4 The irrational state that occurs in response to extreme anxiety is called:

a Fear.   c Tension.

b Conflict.   d Panic.

5 According to intrapsychic theory, anxiety primarily results when:

a Ego functions emerge into consciousness.

b The superego fails to mediate between the id and the ego.

c The id and the superego are in conflict.

d Ego defenses are activated.

6 Which one of the following events did Freud consider prototypical of separation anxiety?

a Birth process.   c Moving out of the home.

b Going to school.   d Death of a loved one.

7 According to interpersonal theory, anxiety is *primarily* conveyed between the infant and the mothering one through:

a Hand gestures.   c Empathic linkage.

b Nonverbal communication.   d Verbal messages.

8 The purpose of mental mechanisms is to do *all but which one* of the following?

a Bring intrapsychic conflicts into consciousness.

b Provide the system with a means to regain homeokinesis.

c Protect the individual from threatening aspects of reality.

d Help maintain the individual's biological integrity.

9 Coping mechanisms *differ* from other mental mechanisms in that they are:

a Used to reduce tension.   c Reality oriented.

b Always unconscious.   d Used to relieve anxiety.

10 Which one of the following coping measures is *most* effective in dealing with stress and anxiety?

a Pleading illness.   c Talking.

b Problem solving.   d Exercising.

11 Making up for a failure or deficiency by emphasizing an asset is a definition of which one of the following ego defense mechanisms?

a Identification.   c Denial.

b Reaction formation.   d Compensation.

12 Mildred left her employer's office feeling hurt and angry that she had been refused a desired and expected promotion. Unable to express her feelings directly, she spent the rest of the day responding impatiently and angrily to her fellow workers. Mildred is probably using the ego defense mechanism of:

a Projection.   c Isolation.

b Sublimation.   d Displacement.

13 Persons who hoard every little thing, much as they withheld their feces in the anal stage of development, are using which one of the following ego defenses?

a Sublimation. c Undoing.
b Fixation. d Introjection.

14 Which one of the following ego defenses is operating when a psychotic person replaces his identity with that of another person?

a Identification. c Denial.
b Reaction formation. d Introjection.

15 The morning after overhearing her parents talking about getting a divorce and arguing over her custody, Sue Ellen awoke and was unable to hear. Physical examination revealed that there was no organic reason for her deafness. Sue Ellen is probably using which adaptive measure to deal with the stress of her parents' impending separation?

a Reaction formation. c Conversion.
b Selective inattention. d Apathy.

16 The ego defense mechanism of isolation is similar to which one of the following security operations?

a Selective inattention. c Preoccupation.
b Somnolent detachment. d Apathy.

17 Sheila is a client on a psychiatric ward. She sits in the corner of the dayroom staring into space, deep in her own thoughts, twirling her hair with her fingers. She is using which one of the following security operations?

a Selective inattention. c Preoccupation.
b Somnolent detachment. d Apathy.

18 Which one of the following mechanisms involves the conscious and purposeful dismissal from awareness of stressful and unpleasant thoughts, feelings, and impulses?

a Suppression. c Isolation.
b Repression. d Denial.

19 Which one of the following mental mechanisms is considered the *healthiest and most effective* adaptation to anxiety?

a Long-term coping mechanisms. c Ego defense mechanisms.
b Short-term coping mechanisms. d Security operations.

20 Long-term coping mechanisms are characterized by which one of the following?

a Seeking immediate relief from anxiety.
b Avoiding conflictual situations.
c Confronting the source of anxiety.
d Dealing with feelings of panic.

13

Biological factors influencing mental health and mental illness

INTRODUCTION

It is generally believed and accepted that the development of mental illness is very complex and probably the result of several factors. In addition to psychosocial, cultural, and environmental factors, the knowledgeable nurse "must become familiar with the growing evidence that points to biological factors as major determinants in the development of mental illness." * However, for one to accept a biological explanation of mental illness, one must assume that an individual's biological development is affected by genetic, biochemical, and neuroanatomical factors that predispose that individual to the development of mental illness. By the same token, one can also assume that the development of mental health is also affected by these same biological factors.

Initial findings from family, twin, adoption, and genetic linkage studies have strongly suggested that genetics plays a significant role in the development of schizophrenia. With the widespread use of psychotropic agents in the treatment of various forms of mental illness, there has been renewed interest in the contribution biochemicals make to the development of mental illness in general and to depression and manic states in particular. Technological advances in recent years have made it feasible to explore, while the client is still alive and can benefit from treatment, the neuroanatomical factors that may play a part in the development of both functional and organic mental disorders.

The exercises in this chapter are designed to help you develop a beginning understanding of some of these biological factors and the role they are believed to play in the development of mental illness.

---

*From Taylor CM: Mereness' essentials of psychiatric nursing, ed 13, St Louis, 1990, The CV Mosby Co, chap 13.

1. To describe the contributions made by leading theorists to our current knowledge of biological factors affecting the development of mental illness.
2. To match genetic findings to their respective genetic studies.
3. To review the dopamine and catecholamine hypotheses.
4. To identify the functions of three brain-imaging procedures.

1 Listed below are the names of five leading theorists who have contributed to our knowledge about biological influences on the development of mental illness. In the space provided, briefly state the role each one played.

a J. Charcot

b S. Freud

c F. Kallman

d A. Carlsson and M. Lindqvist

2 Studies in psychiatric genetics attempt to identify genetic factors influencing the development of various mental disorders. Listed below are ten findings that have been revealed from family, twin, adoption, and/or genetic linkage studies. Match the findings to the relevant study by placing a check in the appropriate column. The first one has been filled in to help you get started.

Findings	Studies			
	Family	Twin	Adoption	Genetic linkage
1. Identical twins develop mental illness more often than do fraternal twins or siblings.	☐	☑	☐	☐
2. Blood relatives of mentally ill persons are more likely to inherit predisposing genes to mental illness.	☐	☐	☐	☐
3. Children separated at birth from their mentally ill parents develop mental illness more often than children separated at birth from biological parents who are not mentally ill.	☐	☐	☐	☐
4. The incidence of schizophrenia in the children of schizophrenic parents is higher than in children whose parents are not schizophrenic and is even higher among identical twins of schizophrenic parents.	☐	☐	☐	☐
5. In children separated from their parents at birth, the incidence of schizophrenia is greater in children whose biological parents are schizophrenic than in children whose biological parents are not schizophrenic.	☐	☐	☐	☐
6. Abnormally functioning genes have been identified in persons suffering from certain types of mental illness.	☐	☐	☐	☐
7. The incidence of schizophrenia is higher in close relations than in the general population who is not related by blood.	☐	☐	☐	☐
8. Fraternal twins or siblings have the same probability of developing mental illness as their parents.	☐	☐	☐	☐
9. The incidence of children's developing schizophrenia is greater when both parents have been diagnosed schizophrenic than when only one parent is schizophrenic.	☐	☐	☐	☐
10. Adopted children whose biological parents are mentally ill have a greater probability of developing mental illness than adopted children of biological parents who are not mentallly ill.	☐	☐	☐	☐

3 Symptoms of mental illness have been identified with neurotransmitters, natural chemicals that function in transmitting nerve impulses to the brain. Two of the most widely known hypotheses linking neurotransmitters and mental illness are the dopamine and catecholamine hypotheses. In the space provided, briefly describe each of these hypotheses.

   a Dopamine hypothesis

   b Catecholamine hypothesis

4 Among the recent advances into the study of biological factors influencing mental health and mental illness are brain studies. Several brain-imaging procedures used in these studies include computed tomography (CT), positron emission tomography (PET), and magnetic resonance imaging (MRI). Some of these procedures are used to assess the presence of organic brain disease, while others have been used to link major mental illnesses to abnormalities in the brain. Listed below are twelve functions that may be attributed to one or more of these three brain-imaging procedures. Read each function and place a check in the appropriate column. The first one has been filled in to help you get started.

Functions	Brain-imaging procedures		
	CT	PET	MRI
1. Assesses organic brain dysfunction.	☑	☑	☑
2. Computes thousands of X rays of the brain	☐	☐	☐
3. Produces a three-dimensional brain image.	☐	☐	☐
4. Allows visualization of several aspects of brain functioning simultaneously.	☐	☐	☐
5. Permits examination of the brain structure.	☐	☐	☐
6. Allows for study of the size of the brain.	☐	☐	☐
7. Identifies brain impairment.	☐	☐	☐
8. Visualizes abnormalities in brain structure.	☐	☐	☐
9. Studies neurochemical and metabolic changes, blood flow, and electrical activity in the brain.	☐	☐	☐
10. Examines the density of designated areas of the brain.	☐	☐	☐
11. Visualizes gross pathology in the brain.	☐	☐	☐
12. Measures physiologic and biochemical functions in brain tissue.	☐	☐	☐

DIRECTIONS: Select the *best* response. (Answers appear in the Appendix.)

1 Immediately following the fall of the Greek and Roman civilizations, the cause of mental illness was largely attributed to:

   a Chemical disturbances in the brain.

   b Religious, mystical, and superstitious factors.

   c Genetic predispositions.

   d Hereditary and environmental factors.

2 Which one of the following occurred in the seventeenth and eighteenth centuries and led to a better understanding of the cause of mental illness?

   a Religious fervor.   **c** Scientific methodology.

   b Political upheaval.   **d** Humanitarian movement.

3 Neurological research into the causes of mental disorders was *first* inspired by the work of:

   a J. Charcot.   **c** M. Lindqvist.

   b S. Freud.   **d** F. Kallman.

4 Which one of the following men was *best* known for his twin studies in the search for the cause of schizophrenia?

   a S. Freud.   **c** A. Carlsson.

   b J. Charcot.   **d** F. Kallman.

5 Recent technological advances have led to the use of new research methods into the cause of mental illness. PET (positron emission tomography) involves which one of the following?

   a Brain-imaging procedures.   **c** Split-brain procedures.

   b Genetic transmission studies.   **d** Neuroendocrine studies.

6 Which of the following methodologies are commonly used in the field of psychiatric genetics?

   a Family studies.   **c** Adoption studies.

   b Twin studies.   **d** All of the above.

7 Which one of the following methodologies has the *most* potential for separating the influences of heredity and environment in studies into the incidence of mental illness?

   a Genetic linkage studies.   **c** Adoption studies.

   b Family studies.   **d** Twin studies.

8 Amino acids, biogenic amines, and neuropeptides are all examples of:

   a Neurotransmitters.   **c** Hormones.

   b Endocrines.   **d** Neurohormones.

9 Which one of the following activity levels of dopamine in the central nervous system characterizes the dopamine hypothesis?

   a Diminished activity.   **c** Imbalance of activity.

   b Overactivity.   **d** Absence of activity.

10 The tricyclics and monoamine oxidase inhibitors are thought to relieve symptoms of depression through their effect on:

a Norepinephrine.   c Histamine.

b Acetylcholine.   d Serotonin.

11 The overactivity observed in manic states is thought to be related to which one of the following levels of catecholamine?

a Diminished catecholamine.   c Elevated catecholamine.

b Lack of catecholamine.   d Excess catecholamine.

12 Which part of the brain plays a major role in controlling the secretion of hormones that affect neural functioning?

a Cerebellum.   c Hypothalamus.

b Thalamus.   d Medulla.

13 Low platelet monoamine oxidase, viral and immunologic deficits, and elevated serum creatine phosphokinase are all biochemical factors believed to affect the incidence of which one of the following mental illnesses?

a Manic states.   c Schizophrenia.

b Depressive states.   d Anxiety disorders.

14 Which one of the following methodologies would be useful in assessing the presence of organic brain dysfunction?

a Computed tomography.   c Magnetic resonance imaging.

b Positron emission tomography.   d All of the above.

15 Symptoms of mental illness may result from which of the following physical problems?

a Encephalitis.   c Brain damage.

b Toxins in the blood.   d All of the above.

14 Cultural factors influencing mental health and mental illness

INTRODUCTION

The United States has always been a culturally pluralistic society. However, it has only been since the 1940s that there has been an increased awareness that ethnicity, gender, and socioeconomic status have influenced society's perception of mental health and mental illness. In addition, it has only been in the last few years that this awareness is being translated into action on the part of health care professionals. Utilizing the nursing process as a framework for nursing care, nurses are combining holistic and individualized care when they assess and collect data about the client's culture, sexual orientation, and socioeconomic situation. With an increased understanding of the total client, the nurse is in a better position to develop more culturally appropriate nursing diagnoses. At the same time, planning, implementing, and evaluating nursing care are more accurate and more meaningful when they are based on an understanding of the client's culturally determined attitudes, beliefs, values, and customs.

"The quality of psychiatric nursing care cannot help but be enhanced when the nurse is aware of the cultural factors that help shape the society's definitions of mental health and mental illness and its choice of mental health treatment."* The exercises in this chapter are designed to help you develop a beginning understanding of selected cultural factors that have relevance for nursing care.

OBJECTIVES

1. To differentiate among selected culturally related terminology.
2. To develop a tool to be used in assessing a client's cultural characteristics.
3. To describe nursing interventions based on an understanding of cultural characteristics.

---

*From Taylor CM: Mereness' essentials of psychiatric nursing, ed 13, St. Louis, 1990, The CV Mosby Co, Chap 14

1 Listed below are eight culturally related terms and eight definitions, one for each term. Match each term with the appropriate definition by placing the number of each definition in the space provided by each culturally related term.

Definition	Term
1. The sum of a society's meanings, expectations, and understandings that characterize a given society's way of life.	___ Cultural norms
	___ Cultural sensitivity
2. The values and beliefs that characterize a given society.	___ Cultural stereotyping
3. Behavior that violates the dominant values and beliefs of a given society.	___ Culture
	___ Deviance
4. Exaggerated beliefs about members of a specific cultural group.	___ Ethnic group
5. Understanding and awareness of the ethnic determinants of another's behavior.	___ Gender
	___ Social drift
6. Racially, geographically, or historically related group with a common and distinct culture.	
7. Phenomenon whereby mentally ill persons experience social disadvantages.	
8. Classification of a person's sex.	

2 List below at least ten questions that you might ask when assessing a client's cultural orientation. The first one has been filled in to help you get started.

a. In what country were you born?

b.

c.

d.

e.

f.

g.

h.

i.

j.

3 Listed below are six characteristics reflecting cultural diversity among different clients. For each one, in the space provided briefly describe a nursing implication. One nursing implication for clients with an Italian heritage has been filled in to help you get started. You should be able to think of a second one for Italian clients.

Cultural characteristics of clients	Nursing implication
1. Italian: continuous emotional involvement among all members of the extended family is a norm.	Show understanding when a hospitalized client is visited by multiple family members while setting necessary limits on numbers.
2. Chinese: modest, reserved, and noncomplaining.	
3. Puerto Rican: common belief among some persons that spirits have the power to influence one's life.	
4. Black American: Hostile, suspicious, and reluctant to talk about themselves to nonblack caregivers.	
5. Asian and Hispanic: Appears to seek help from mental health professionals less often than do white American clients.	
6. American Indian and black American: Appear to drop out of treatment prematurely.	

DIRECTIONS: Select the *best* response. (Answers appear in the Appendix.)

1 The nursing specialty that *most* specifically bases nursing intervention on an understanding of beliefs and practices of different ethnic groups is:
   a Psychiatric nursing.
   b Community mental health nursing.
   c Transcultural nursing.
   d Mental health nursing.

2 Cultural norms refer to which one of the following?
   a The sum total of a society's meanings, expectations, and understandings.
   b The values and beliefs that characterize a given society.
   c The exaggerated beliefs about members of a cultural group.
   d All of the above.

3 Which one of the following results from labeling members of a society deviant?
   a Helping to unify the controlling social group.
   b Placing persons violating cultural norms outside the ruling social group.
   c Allowing the dominant social group to affirm the rightness of its values.
   d All of the above.

4 Deviance labeling generally leads to *all but which one* of the following?
   a Racism.
   b Sexism.
   c Feminism.
   d Classism.

5 In an effort to develop cultural sensitivity toward clients, nurses must be cautious about:
   a Reverting to cultural stereotyping.
   b Losing sight of each client's uniqueness.
   c Overgeneralizing about all clients of a particular ethnic group.
   d All of the above.

6 The culturally aware nurse knows that shyness, modesty, and introverted behaviors are considered virtues by which one of the following ethnic groups?
   a White Americans.
   b Puerto Ricans.
   c Italians.
   d Chinese.

7 Continuous involvement among all members of the extended family is the norm in which one of the following ethnic groups?
   a Swedish Americans.
   b Anglo-Saxon Americans.
   c Italian Americans.
   d Black Americans.

8 Persons with a Puerto Rican heritage who believe in spiritualism may be mistakenly diagnosed as psychotic and said to be experiencing:
   a Delusions.
   b Illusions.
   c Hallucinations.
   d Compulsions.

9 Recognizing that some black Americans tend to hesitate to talk about themselves and reveal their innermost feelings and thoughts, the nurse needs to be particularly:
   a Sympathetic.
   b Patient.
   c Consistent.
   d Persistent.

10 Which one of the following cultural groups tends to seek and follow through with professional mental health care the *most*?

    a Asian Americans.
    c Black Americans.
    b Hispanic Americans.
    d White Americans.

11 The nurse can be *most* helpful with clients who have a tendency to drop out of treatment prematurely by doing which one of the following?

    a Utilizing short-term crisis-oriented therapy.
    b Referring clients for psychotherapy.
    c Making sure clients have a sufficient supply of medications on hand.
    d Learning clients' address and phone number early in treatment.

12 Gender appears to be a factor influencing the nature of mental health problems. Studies suggest that men, more than women, tend to experience which one of the following disorders *most*?

    a Depressive reactions.
    c Eating disorders.
    b Phobic disorders.
    d Alcohol abuse.

13 In general, men tend to seek out mental health services less frequently than women. This is probably because they perceive such actions as:

    a Too time-consuming.
    c Too expensive.
    b A sign of weakness.
    d A waste of time.

14 The opposing view to the phenomenon known as *social drift* states that:

    a Socioeconomic disadvantages contribute to increased stress and the onset of mental illness.
    b Mentally ill persons experience socioeconomic disadvantages as a consequence of their illness.
    c Prevalence of mental illness among the socially disadvantaged is genetically based.
    d None of the above.

15 Which of the following questions would be appropriate to ask when assessing a client's cultural orientation?

    a "How do you feel about being touched by a stranger?"
    b "What languages do you speak, read, or write?"
    c "Who constitutes your immediate family?"
    d All of the above.

Section three word games and section exercises

1 Matching: Historical perspective

DIRECTIONS: Listed below are the names of fifteen persons who have contributed significantly to the fields of psychiatry and psychiatric–mental health nursing. Also listed are their contributions. Match the person with the contribution by placing the number of the contribution in the space provided by the contributor. The first one has been filled in to help you get started. (The solution appears in the Appendix.)

Contributions	Contributors
1. First theorist to identify stress as a factor in causing disease.	___ Becker
2. Identified the *eight ages of man*.	_1_ Cannon
3. Took issue with the practice of labeling socially deviant behaviors mental illness.	___ Carlsson
4. Identified criteria of positive mental health.	___ Charcot
5. Pioneered the study of the biochemical model of stress and adaptation.	___ Erikson
6. Investigated the role of genetics in the development of mental illness through the study of identical twins.	___ Freud
7. Focused on the effect cultural norms have on psychological development.	___ Horney
8. Initiated discussion of general systems theory.	___ Jahoda
9. Introduced the psychosexual theory of personality development.	___ Kallman
10. Identified the phenomenon of labeling as deviant one who violates cultural norms.	___ Maslow
11. Pioneered work on cognitive development.	___ Piaget
12. Developed the interpersonal theory of psychiatry.	___ Selye
13. Introduced, with Lindqvist, the dopamine hypothesis of schizophrenia.	___ Sullivan
14. Conducted early research into the cause of nervous and mental disorders.	___ Szasz
15. Introduced the *hierarchy of needs* theory.	___ von Bertalanffy

2 Fill-in: Mental mechanisms

DIRECTIONS: Using the definitions provided, fill in the word list with selected *mental mechanisms* discussed in the text. (The solution appears in the Appendix.)

Definitions	Word List
A Unconsciously redirecting anxiety-producing impulses into acceptable channels	_ _ _ _ _ _ M _ _ _ _ _
B Expressing conflicts through physical symptoms for which there is no organic basis	_ _ _ _ _ E _ _ _ _ _
C Engaging in certain activities to cancel out unconscious anxiety-producing thoughts	_ N _ _ _ _ _ _
D Halting emotional development at a point in time	_ _ _ _ _ T _ _ _
E Recalling a painful event without experiencing the pain	_ _ _ _ _ A _ _ _ _
F Involuntarily refusing to acknowledge reality	_ _ _ _ _ _ L
G Dealing directly with anxiety rather than avoiding it (two words)	_ _ _ _ _ _ _ M _ _ _ _ _ _
H Reverting to behaviors more typical of an earlier age	_ _ _ _ _ E _ _ _ _
I Manifesting consuming interest in something to exclude anxiety-producing reality	_ _ _ _ _ C _ _ _ _ _ _
J Exhibiting extreme indifference to an event that would usually elicit anxiety	_ _ _ _ H _
K Discharging emotions associated with a subject on an entirely different one	_ _ _ _ _ A _ _ _ _ _
L Unconsciously justifying one's activities with excuses	_ _ _ _ _ N _ _ _ _ _ _ _
M Using a seemingly neutral object to represent a conflictual one	_ _ _ _ _ _ _ I _ _ _ _ _ _
N Intentionally dismissing troubling thoughts from consciousness	_ _ _ _ _ S _ _ _
O Emphasizing an asset to make up for a weakness	_ _ M _ _ _ _ _ _ _ _
P Involuntarily excluding thoughts from consciousness	_ _ _ _ _ S _ _ _

113

3 Crosshatch

DIRECTIONS: Fit the seventy-seven words listed below into the proper boxes. The words read left to right or top to bottom, one letter per box. ADAPTATIONS has been entered to give you a starting point. (The solution appears in the Appendix.)

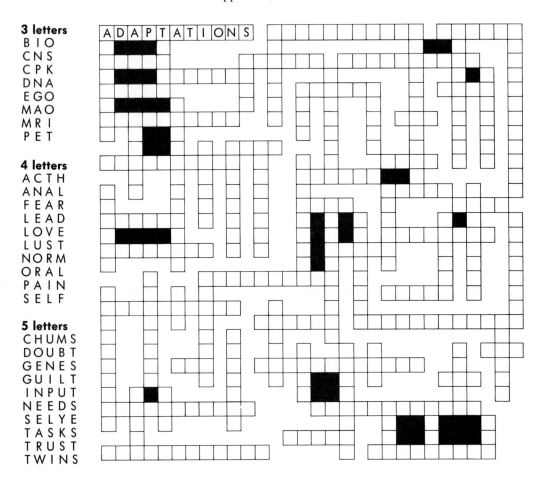

3 letters
BIO
CNS
CPK
DNA
EGO
MAO
MRI
PET

4 letters
ACTH
ANAL
FEAR
LEAD
LOVE
LUST
NORM
ORAL
PAIN
SELF

5 letters
CHUMS
DOUBT
GENES
GUILT
INPUT
NEEDS
SELYE
TASKS
TRUST
TWINS

6 letters
APATHY
COPING
CRISIS
DENIAL
ENERGY
ETHNIC
GENDER
MASLOW
OUTPUT
PIAGET
RACISM
STRESS
VALUES

7 letters
CHARCOT
ERIKSON
INFANCY
KALLMAN

8 letters
ADOPTION
AUTONOMY
CONCEPTS
DEVIANCE
DOPAMINE
EMPATHIC
GENETICS
LABELING
MINORITY
SECURITY
STRESSOR
SULLIVAN

9 letters
ISOLATION
WHOLENESS

10 letters
ENDOCRINES
INITIATIVE
MECHANISMS
NEGENTROPY
REPRESSION
STAGNATION
SUBSYSTEMS
THROUGHPUT

11 letters
ADAPTATIONS
CHROMOSOMES
OMNIPOTENCE

12 letters
HOMEOKINESIS
INTRAPSYCHIC
INTROJECTION
NEUROPEPTIDE
PERMEABILITY
SATISFACTION
STEREOTYPING

114

4 Quote-a-crostic

DIRECTIONS: Using cues on the left, fill in the words in the list on the right. Transfer each letter in the word list to the corresponding numbered square in the puzzle grid on p. 116. Shaded squares in the grid represent the ends of words. Work back and forth between grid and word list until both are completed. (Note the letters and consecutive numbers that have been entered in the grid to help in location of words.) The completed grid will be a quotation relevant to Section III of the text. The source of the quote and its author are spelled out in the boxed-in letters in the word list. The first word in the list has been filled in to help you get started. (The solution appears in the Appendix.)

Cues

Word List

A Subjective phenomena

<u>S</u> <u>T</u> <u>R</u> <u>E</u> <u>S</u> <u>S</u>
39 145 81 177 54 99

B Stigmatized

___ ___ ___ |___| ___ ___ ___
107 33 143 53 93 158 67

C Period characterized by oedipal
conflict (two words)

___ ___ ___ ___ ___ ___ ___
42 181 92 5 76 14 32

___ ___ ___ ___ ___
173 10 166 87 144

D MAO inhibitors:
_____ elevators

___ |___| ___ ___
116 180 128 141

E Erogenous area (two words)

___ ___ ___ ___   ___ ___ |___| ___
21 134 117 13   50 59 149 182

F Negative or positive

___ ___ ___ |___| ___ ___ ___ ___
137 175 147 130 78 25 88 115

G One of the neuropeptides

___ ___ ___ ___ ___ ___ |___| ___ ___
148 52 105 95 12 174 165 161 154

H Tool in early childhood

___ ___ ___ |___| ___
120 66 146 71 4

I Toxic substance

___ ___ |___| ___
77 91 153 57

115

1 V	2 J	3 N	4 H	5 C	6 P	■	7 P	8 K	9 V	■	10 C	11 V	12 G	■	13 E	14 C	15 Q	16 W	■		
17 R	18 V	19 S	■	20 T	21 E	22 J	■	23 P	24 U	25 F	26 N	■	27 Q	28 P	29 L	■	30 P	31 N	32 C	33 B	34 W	35 U
■	36 J	37 S	38 K	39 A S	40 P	41 T	42 C	43 N	44 Q	45 V	■	46 N	47 J	48 Q	49 R	50 E	51 P	52 G	53 B	54 A S	
55 J	56 M	57 I	■	58 P	59 E	60 J	61 V	62 Q	63 K	■	64 U	65 V	66 H	67 B	■	68 N	69 M	70 J	71 H	72 K	73 S
74 R	75 Q	76 C	77 I	78 F	79 P	80 O	81 A R	82 N	■	83 W	84 J	85 T	86 P	87 C	■	88 F	89 P	90 U	91 I	92 C	93 B
94 N	95 G	96 W	97 P	98 V	■	99 A S	100 N	101 W	■	102 P	103 J	104 L	105 G	■	106 N	107 B	108 T	■	109 J	110 K	111 S
112 M	113 N	114 U	115 F	■	116 D	117 E	118 Q	119 P	■	120 H	121 T	122 P	123 R	124 J	125 L	126 Q	■	127 L	128 D	129 J	130 F
131 S	■	132 N	133 Q	134 E	135 P	■	136 N	137 F	■	138 V	139 J	140 S	141 D	142 K	■	143 B	144 C	145 A T	146 H	147 F	148 G	149 E
■	150 R	151 K	152 P	■	153 I	154 G	155 U	■	156 Q	157 M	158 B	■	159 J	160 Q	161 G	162 K	163 S	■	164 W	165 G	166 C	167 P
168 Q	169 M	170 O	■	171 P	172 J	173 C	174 G	175 F	176 O	177 A E	178 M	■	179 Q	180 D	■	181 C	182 E	183 W	■		

Cues—cont'd

J Violation of cultural norms (two words)

__ __ __ __ __ __ __
22　2　70　124　47　36　159

__ __ __ __ |60| __ __ __
55　103　109　172　60　84　139　129

K Health

__ __ __ __ __ |151| __ __
38　110　8　72　162　151　63　142

L Signal, as in anxiety

__ __ __ |125|
127　104　29　125

M Identified criteria for positive mental health

|112| __ __ __ __ __
112　56　157　69　178　169

N Negative outcomes of task autonomy (three words)

__ __ __ __ __　__ __ __
31　100　3　46　43　106　68　26

__ __ |113| __ __
82　136　113　94　132

O Molecule carrying genetic information (abb.)

|170| __ __
170　176　80

Word List—cont'd

P Sullivan's contribution (two
   words)
      `51` 58 122 89 102   —

      40 30 23 135 79 86 7 119

      167 171 97 28 152 6

Q Body's response to life-threatening situations
      15 75 126 160 `156` 133 44

      27 62 118 48 168 179

R Solace for someone preoccupied
   with cleanliness
      74 49 123 `150` 17

S Revert to outgrown behaviors
      111 37 `163` 140 19 131 73

T Sometimes relieves anxiety
      108 41 `121` 85 20

U Male or female
      64 `35` 114 155 24 90

V Concept related to the concept of
   nonsummativity
      138 18 65 9 61 1 11 98 `45`

W Piaget, Selye, and von Bertalanffy, for example
      16 96 34 101 183 `164` 83

15 | *Individuals with thought disorders*

INTRODUCTION

Individuals with thought disorders are generally given the medical diagnosis of schizophrenia, "...one of the *functional psychoses*. This term describes those mental illnesses for which there is no demonstrable organic disease or intellectual deficit and where the illness is all-pervasive, affecting all dimensions of the person's existence." *

To be diagnosed schizophrenic, one must be functioning at a level below that which one had previously achieved. In addition, characteristic behaviors such as delusions, associative looseness (derailment), hallucinations, apathy, ambivalence, inappropriate affect/behavior, withdrawal from reality, autistic thinking, and psychomotor retardation and/or overactivity must be evident for a 6-month period or more.

Schizophrenia is a long-term disorder, with symptomatology commonly first manifested in late adolescence or young adulthood, whose cause is not conclusively agreed upon. Theorists suggest that a combination of genetic, physiological, biochemical, and/or emotional factors may predispose an individual to the development of a thought disorder.

Genetic studies such as Kallman's with identical twins have suggested that schizophrenia may be inherited. Various brain studies of schizophrenic individuals have demonstrated abnormal glucose utilization and decreased brain size, suggesting a physiological cause and/or effect to schizophrenia. Biochemical studies such as Carlsson and Lindqvist's dopamine hypothesis of schizophrenia may reveal how and why psychotropic agents are effective in controlling symptomatology seen in thought disorders.

Of all the factors, however, the emotional ones seem to provide the greatest direction for the carrying out of nursing care with clients with a thought disorder. Sullivan's interpersonal theory of psychiatry proposes that persons with a thought disorder have a predominantly bad-me/not-me self-concept resulting from a

---

*From Taylor CM: Mereness' essentials of psychiatric nursing, ed 13, St Louis, 1990, The CV Mosby Co, chap 15.

combination of negative reflected appraisals, excessive anxiety, and unmet needs. Patterns of interaction between an individual and his or her significant other in the early years of the individual's development were often characterized by double-bind communication. According to Bateson, double-bind communication involves the giving of two contradictory messages simultaneously by one person, contributing to anxiety and confusion in the individual. Repetitive experiences of this type with significant persons throughout the formative years interfere with the development of a healthy self-concept and reinforce the early learning that relating is painful and best avoided.

Erikson's cultural theory of development states that an individual proceeds through eight stages of life. Associated with each stage is a culturally determined task that is identified as a challenge to be met and mastered. A person with a thought disorder is believed to have experienced traumas in infancy that interfere with the successful mastery of the first developmental task of trust. Inconsistently met needs, unpredictability, covert and overt expressions of indifference, and lack of love from parenting figures contribute to the negative outcome of mistrust and lay the foundation for nontrusting relationships with others in subsequent years. In addition, because each age builds on earlier ages, difficulty mastering trust in infancy interferes with the mastery of subsequent tasks in later stages of life if the individual continues to be exposed to negative life experiences.

Both the interpersonal and cultural theories stress that persons with a thought disorder have experienced personality disruption during infancy. Because individuals are essentially dependent at this time, they are most vulnerable and lack the tools to deal effectively with painful and anxiety-producing situations. If these anxiety-producing situations continue to predominate during the formative years, personality development will be further impaired. Subsequent stressors in adolescence and adulthood can be overwhelming and precipitate a profound psychotic response in the form of a thought disorder as the individual tries to cope ineffectively with life's challenges.

With this theoretical understanding, nurses can intervene therapeutically and help clients with thought disorders learn healthier adaptations. Nurses can involve clients in therapeutic nurse-client relationships and show them that not all relating is anxiety provoking and best avoided. Nurses can provide clients with corrective experiences and help them develop more positive perceptions of themselves. Nurses can also assist clients to renegotiate the developmental tasks they may have failed to master.

In developing a plan of care for the individual with a thought disorder, the nurse utilizes the five phases of the nursing process. Beginning with assessment, the nurse observes behavior and collects data. One or more nursing diagnoses are then identified and the presenting problems and possible etiological factors determined. Subsequently, a plan of nursing action is formulated, implemented, and, ultimately, evaluated for its effectiveness.

The exercises in this chapter are designed to help you understand the nature of thought disorders, to apply selected phases of the nursing process to the care of individuals with thought disorders, and to begin to develop some understanding about the use of antipsychotic medications in the treatment of individuals with thought disorders.

OBJECTIVES

1. To categorize behaviors exhibited by individuals with thought disorders according to the five subtypes of schizophrenia.
2. To analyze behaviors using interpersonal and cultural theories.
3. To apply selected phases of the nursing process to clinical situations.
4. To identify the action, dosage, administration, contraindications, precautions, idiosyncrasies, side and adverse effects, and nursing implications relevant to the use of antipsychotic medications.

EXERCISES

1 People with thought disorders are given a medical diagnosis of schizophrenia. In addition, they are further classified according to subtypes, depending on the predominant behavioral patterns exhibited at the time of diagnosis. The following exercise lists fifteen behaviors commonly observed in schizophrenic persons and the five subtypes of schizophrenia. Read and categorize each behavior, placing a check in the box or boxes in the appropriate columns. The first one has been filled in to help you get started.

| | Subtypes of schizophrenia | | | | |
Behaviors	Disorganized	Catatonic	Paranoid	Chronic undiff.	Residual
1. Soiling self.	☑	☑	☐	☑	☐
2. Maintaining motionless state.	☐	☐	☐	☐	☐
3. Responding with bursts of overactivity.	☐	☐	☐	☐	☐
4. Accusing others falsely.	☐	☐	☐	☐	☐
5. Exhibiting flat, blunt affect.	☐	☐	☐	☐	☐
6. Isolating self from others, but exhibiting no overt psychotic signs.	☐	☐	☐	☐	☐
7. Masturbating openly.	☐	☐	☐	☐	☐
8. Expressing grandiose delusions.	☐	☐	☐	☐	☐
9. Projecting fears and suspicions onto others.	☐	☐	☐	☐	☐
10. Giggling inappropriately.	☐	☐	☐	☐	☐
11. Experiencing auditory hallucinations.	☐	☐	☐	☐	☐
12. Expressing ideas of persecution.	☐	☐	☐	☐	☐
13. Exhibiting psychomotor retardation.	☐	☐	☐	☐	☐
14. Avoiding social situations.	☐	☐	☐	☐	☐
15. Manifesting pressured speech.	☐	☐	☐	☐	☐

2 Read the following situation and then complete the exercises as directed.
SITUATION: Penny Porter, a 25-year-old white, single woman, was brought to the admitting office by her mother. Mrs. Porter expressed frustration over

her daughter's recent behavior, saying, (1) *"Last month Penny stopped going to her job and sat at home talking to herself. She wouldn't talk to me."* Penny's mother continued, "And, as if that wasn't enough, (2) *she has gotten so suspicious. She says that I hate her and am trying to poison her. She refuses to eat with me. The only time she goes out is to buy herself some food, which she eats immediately. She won't share anything with me. I'm an old lady. I don't deserve to be treated this way."* Mrs. Porter sat back in her chair and glared angrily at her daughter, who appeared not to notice anything that had been said. Further information elicited in the interview was that Mr. Porter had walked out on his wife and daughter when Penny was an infant. Penny was raised in a series of foster homes while her mother went out to work. (3) *Penny had no friends in school. She preferred solitary activities such as reading and watching television to interacting socially with her peers.* (4) *Mrs. Porter recalled that Penny had to wear faded and mended clothing belonging to other children in the foster homes, and she was embarrassed to go to school where she felt "different" from the other children.* When Penny graduated from high school, she returned to her mother's house and worked at a variety of unskilled jobs. However, because of her uncommunicative and aloof manner, she never stayed in any job very long. (5) *After being terminated in a job, she would come home crying, saying how bad she was for not being better able to help her mother. She would punish herself by standing in a corner for long hours, just as she had been punished as a child.*

Penny Porter was admitted to the psychiatric service for observation and treatment. In the unit (6) *she sat alone, talking to herself. She usually sat facing the door, and her eyes followed all who entered. If approached from the rear, she would whirl around snarling, "Don't you sneak up on me!"* (7) *She took no responsibility for her personal hygiene and appeared disheveled unless staff intervened. When encouraged to choose what she would wear, she became anxious and unable to make a decision.* (8) *Initially she refused to follow any suggestions and often did the opposite of what was expected of her.* (9) *Later she would find a remote area, sit on the floor, close her eyes, and chant in a loud voice devoid of feeling, "Dear God, dear God. Forgive her for her sins. She is so bad. Punish her, God. Send her to Hell. Forgive her, God, dear God, dear God."* (10) *In addition to referring to herself as "she" and "her," there were times when Penny would not respond to her name, saying, "Penny? Who is Penny? Call me 'Nobody.'"* (11) *Penny was given clay to mold but had a hard time concentrating on even the simplest craft activity, such as making an ashtray out of clay. She never completed anything she started. Even with encouragement she expressed feelings of inadequacy saying, "Oh, I could never do that. It would never be good enough to suit Mother."* (12) *At meals she continued to experience episodes of suspiciousness, accusing staff of trying to poison her "just like my mother."*

a Using Sullivan's interpersonal theory, briefly speculate on the nature of Penny Porter's relationships with others. Begin with Penny's first significant other, her mother, and trace her relationships with others up to the onset of her psychotic symptoms. (Where possible, use available data such as the father's leaving home when she was an infant. Speculate on the effect this had on Penny and her mother and Penny's subsequent relationships with men.)

b Although it is generally preferable that assessment data in the form of observational material be described in detail, it is also necessary for the nurse to be aware of the commonly used psychiatric terminologies applicable to behaviors manifested by persons with thought disorders. Listed below are fifteen behaviors exhibited by Penny Porter and fifteen psychiatric terms that can be attached to these behaviors. Match the term with the behavior by placing the number of the behavior in the space provided next to the term. The first one has been filled in to help you get started.

Behaviors	Terminology
1. Sitting alone and avoiding all interpersonal contacts.	___ Ambivalence
2. Communicating in hard-to-follow sentences, jumping from one unrelated topic to another.	___ Associative looseness
	___ Auditory hallucinations
3. Expressing an unfounded belief that people are trying to poison her.	___ Autism
	___ Delusions of grandeur
4. Talking out loud when no one else is present.	___ Flat affect
5. Reverting to infantile behaviors that had been outgrown, such as untidiness and soiling herself.	___ Inappropriate affect/ behavior
6. Failing to communicate feelings either in her speech or her facial expression.	___ Mutism
	___ Negativism
7. Appearing deep in her own private thoughts and not sharing them with others.	___ Persecutory delusions
	___ Psychomotor overactivity
8. Expressing the unfounded belief that her body is deteriorating.	___ Psychomotor retardation
9. Growing increasingly inactive, standing or sitting immobile for hours at a time.	___ Regression
10. Refusing to act on suggestions, often responding opposite to what is expected.	___ Somatic delusions
11. Laughing for no apparent reason.	_1_ Withdrawal
12. Becoming increasingly nonverbal, not speaking for weeks at a time.	
13. Experiencing two contradictory feelings simultaneously.	
14. Expressing unfounded beliefs of self-importance.	
15. Exhibiting pressured speech on occasion.	

c In this situation the nurse, using assessment skills, noted that many of the client's behaviors reflect problems with developmental tasks. Refer to the twelve italicized and numbered behaviors in the situation and indicate in the following grid which developmental tasks or negative outcomes of developmental tasks they reflect. Some behaviors may reflect more than one task or outcome. One behavior has been filled in to help you get started. Although you could merely write in the number of the behavior in the space provided, it is recommended that you write out or paraphrase the behavior as in the example.

Developmental tasks/ Negative outcomes	Discussion
1. Trust/mistrust	
2. Autonomy/shame and doubt	
3. Initiative/guilt	
4. Industry/inferiority	
5. Identity/role confusion	
6. Intimacy/isolation	(1) Staying at home and isolating herself from fellow workers and her mother; talking to herself rather than to others.

d Develop a plan of care for Penny Porter. Four pairs of nursing diagnoses and appropriate nursing objectives have been filled in to help focus you on specific areas requiring nursing intervention. Complete the exercise by providing several appropriate nursing actions and outcome criteria for each objective.

Nursing diagnosis	Objective	Nursing actions	Outcome criteria
1. Altered Self-Concept R/T negative reflected appraisals (ANA: 6.3.2) OR Self-Esteem Disturbance R/T negative appraisals (NANDA: 7.1.2).	To help client develop a more positive concept of self.		
2. Altered Self-Care R/T feelings of worthlessness (ANA: 1.3.4) OR Bathing/Hygiene Self-Care Deficit R/T feelings of worthlessness (NANDA: 6.5.2) OR Dressing/Grooming Self-Care Deficit R/T feelings of worthlessness (NANDA: 6.5.3).	To help client assume responsibility for bathing and dressing appropriately.		
3. Altered Social Interaction R/T lack of trust (ANA: 5.7.2) OR Impaired Social Interaction R/T lack of trust (NANDA: 3.1.1).	To help client develop a sense of trust in the nurse.		
4. Altered Thought Processes R/T delusions (ANA: 2.6.2) (NANDA: 8.3).	To help diminish client's delusional thinking.		

3 Complete the following exercises on nursing diagnoses.*

    a Listed below are the eight human processes around which current nursing assessment and diagnoses have been organized according to the ANA Classification of Human Responses of Concern for Psychiatric Mental Health Nursing Practice, Draft IV-R (September 20, 1988). In the space provided identify at least one nursing diagnosis for each human process. Each diagnosis should be relevant to the problems reflected in clients with a thought disorder. Each diagnosis should consist of a problem statement and a possible etiological factor. The first one has been filled in to help you get started.

       1. Activity processes:

          Altered Motor Behavior R/T psychomotor retardation (1.1.2).

      2. Cognition processes:

      3. Ecological processes:

      4. Emotional processes:

      5. Interpersonal processes:

      6. Perception processes:

      7. Physiological processes:

      8. Valuation processes:

---

*See Taylor CM: Mereness' essentials of psychiatric nursing, ed 13, St Louis, 1990, The CV Mosby Co, Appendix D and E, for help in completing these exercises.

b The NANDA Approved Nursing Diagnostic Categories (1988) have been organized around nine categories or patterns. In the space provided identify at least one approved nursing diagnosis for each pattern using the NANDA format. Each diagnosis should be relevant to the problems reflected in clients with a thought disorder. Each diagnosis should consist of a problem statement and a possible etiological factor. The first one has been filled in to help you get started.

1. Pattern 1: Exchanging
   Urinary Retention R/T the toxic effect of antipsychotic medications (1.3.2.2).

2. Pattern 2: Communicating

3. Pattern 3: Relating

4. Pattern 4: Valuing

5. Pattern 5: Choosing

6. Pattern 6: Moving

7. Pattern 7: Perceiving

8. Pattern 8: Knowing

9. Pattern 9: Feeling

4 Learning about medications requires self-discipline, incentive to learn, repetition, and several good source books on medications. In addition to your psychiatric text, you will want to refer to a reputable pharmacology book and, perhaps, the current *Physicians' Desk Reference,* which is generally available on most hospital units as well as in college libraries. If you have already established a useful pattern for learning about medications in other nursing courses, it is hoped you will incorporate your system into the study and learning of psychotropic agents. If you have not, you may find the following exercises useful in helping you develop such a system. It is based on the collection of data on "drug cards." You can develop your own format or use the one suggested here. You can use any size cards convenient for you, but they should be uniform in size to file for future reference. If you own or have access to a personal computer with a printer, you can set up your "cards" on the computer, enter and store your data, and make a hard copy to take to the clinical area for reference. Later, as you gather additional data or are assigned to other clients receiving the same medications, you can update your drug cards without having to recopy all the material previously entered.

Individuals with the medical diagnosis of schizophrenia are often prescribed one of the antipsychotic medications. These agents help control psychotic symptoms and make clients more amenable to other aspects of their treatment program. In this exercise fill in the data on the following drug card for thioridazine (Mellaril), one of the commonly used antipsychotic agents. Use your psychiatric nursing and pharmacology texts to help you complete the exercise.

(Side one)

Generic name: Thioridazine
Trade name: Mellaril

Classification:
Other drugs in this classification:

Action:

Range of daily dosage/route of administration:

Date/client initials/dosage:

Contraindications/precautions:

Drug idiosyncrasies:

(Side two)

Side and adverse effects: Nursing implications for each:

Miscellaneous nursing implications:

Source of data and date:

5 In the technical role, the nurse prepares and administers medications to clients as prescribed by the physician. In addition to dosage and action, the knowledgeable nurse needs to be aware of possible side and toxic effects associated with the use of medications and the appropriate nursing actions that should be taken if they arise. Drowsiness, for example, is an expected, transient side effect accompanying the use of most antipsychotic agents. Knowing this, the nurse will not become alarmed if the client appears drowsy. By the same token, the nurse will not allow the client to use the symptom as an excuse for not participating in a treatment program. Nursing actions in response to drowsiness might include having the client splash his or her face with cold water, drink a cup of coffee, and walk. Clients receiving medications and treated in clinics would be specifically cautioned against driving or engaging in activities requiring mental acuity. In addition, administering the medication at bedtime would be a way to render an annoying side effect therapeutic by helping the client sleep at night. In the following exercise are listed fifteen side or adverse effects associated with the use of antipsychotic agents and ten nursing actions that should be carried out in response to these effects. Match the appropriate nursing action to the side/adverse effect by placing the letter of the action in the space provided next to the side/adverse effect. In this exercise a nursing action may be used in response to more than one side/adverse effect. The first one has been filled in to help you get started.

Side/adverse effects	Nursing actions
1. Agranulocytosis _f_ 2. Akathisia ___ 3. Constipation ___ 4. Convulsions ___ 5. Dry mouth ___ 6. Dystonia ___ 7. Jaundice ___ 8. Leukopenia ___ 9. Ocular changes ___ 10. Orthostatic hypotension ___ 11. Paralytic ileus ___ 12. Photosensitivity ___ 13. Pseudoparkinsonism ___ 14. Tardive dyskinesia ___ 15. Urinary hesitance/ retention ___	a. Administer anticonvulsant medication as ordered. b. Offer fluids, sugarless chewing gum, or hard candy. c. Provide fluids, balanced diet with roughage; use laxatives as necessary. d. Notify physician and withhold medication. e. Report complaints of blurred vision or squinting to the physician and provide periodic eye examinations. f. Check out and report any symptoms of colds or sore throat and see that white blood counts are carried out periodically. g. Protect from rays of the sun by keeping the client in the shade and having client wear a hat and long sleeves. h. Notify physician but do not withhold medication. i. Reassure the client, notify the physician, and administer antiparkinsonism medications as ordered. j. Take client's blood pressure before starting drug and ambulate gradually at any sign of lightheadedness.

TEST ITEMS

DIRECTIONS: Select the *best* response. (Answers appear in the Appendix.)

1 The term *schizophrenia* was first used by:

   a Eugene Bleuler.   c Emil Kraepelin.

   b Jean Charcot.   d Manfred Sakel.

2 The DSM-III published in 1980 was the first diagnostic manual to do which one of the following?

   a Define the many varieties of mental disorders.

   b Analyze the behaviors in mentally ill persons.

   c Assess mentally ill persons holistically.

   d Classify mental disorders systematically.

3 A functional psychosis is one in which there is:

   a No disturbance in the cognitive area.

   b Intellectual deficit and dysfunction.

   c No demonstrable organic disease.

   d Pervasive physiological disturbances.

4 Positive symptoms of schizophrenia refer *most* specifically to behaviors reflecting:

   a Distortions in thinking and perceiving.

   b Functional responses to stress.

   c Disturbances in affect and volition.

   d Dysfunctional interpersonal relationships.

5 Which one of the following symptoms of schizophrenia primarily reflects distortions in form rather than content of thought?

   a Hallucinations.   c Flat affect.

   b Delusions.   d Associative looseness.

6 Which one of the following types of hallucinations is *most* commonly manifested in schizophrenia?

   a Visual.   c Olfactory.

   b Auditory.   d Tactile.

7 Loss of ego boundaries would *most* specifically be manifested by which one of the following?

   a Expressions of worthlessness and low self-esteem.

   b Inability to differentiate between self and the environment.

   c Inability to initiate self-care or work activities.

   d Expressions of self-destructive impulses.

8 Schizophrenia may be categorized into one of several subtypes. A person with the disorganized subtype would generally exhibit which of the following behaviors?

   a Explosive bursts of overactivity and expressions of confused thinking.

   b Loss of animation and a tendency to remain in the same position for long periods.

   c Aggressive acts and false accusations directed at others.

   d Hallucinatory behaviors and open masturbation in front of others.

9 Individuals who exhibit some inappropriate, but not psychotic, behaviors would be classified according to which one of the following subtypes?

   a Residual.   c Catatonic.

   b Undifferentiated.   d Paranoid.

10 A positive prognosis for a person with a thought disorder is *primarily* based on the client's:

a Diagnosis and subtype.

b Willingness to take medications.

c Available resources.

d Prepsychotic personality.

11 Which one of the following would be the *best* example of a *precipitating* factor in the development of schizophrenia?

a Biochemical composition.

b Genetic make-up.

c Stressful event.

d Physiological structure.

12 Which one of the following symptoms reflects endocrine changes that sometimes occur with the use of antipsychotic drugs?

a Dry mouth.

b Weight gain.

c Constipation.

d Hypotension.

13 In response to orthostatic hypotension, the nurse can be *most* helpful to the client by taking which one of the following actions?

a Staying with the client until the hypotensive episode passes.

b Teaching the client to rise slowly before standing.

c Encouraging the client to walk slowly.

d Checking the client's blood pressure at regular intervals.

14 Akathisia is identifiable by which one of the following symptoms?

a Masklike facies.

b Muscle weakness.

c Shuffling gait.

d Neck spasms.

15 The nurse might suspect that a client on Thorazine (chlorpromazine) was developing agranulocytosis if the client complained of:

a Sore throat.

b Blurred vision.

c Constipation.

d Dizziness.

16 If a client on an antipsychotic agent shows signs of tardive dyskinesia, the nurse should take which one of the following actions *immediately?*

a Administer a prn order of an antiparkinsonian drug.

b Notify the physician and withhold the antipsychotic drug.

c Administer the antipsychotic agent and report the symptoms to the physician.

d Reassure the client that the symptoms are transient and will subside shortly.

17 Behaviors observed in thought disorders can be grouped around one of eight human processes. Which of the following behaviors reflect an impairment of the *perception* process?

a Indecisiveness.

b Poor judgment.

c Delusional thinking.

d Hallucinations.

18 Which one of the following physical problems is commonly seen in clients exhibiting psychomotor retardation?

a Weight loss.

b Muscular rigidity.

c Edema.

d Hypotension.

19 Clients' disturbance in volition often requires that the nurse take which one of the following actions?

    a Encourage clients to participate in self-care and/or recreational activities.

    b Give clients positive reflected appraisals for their improved appearance.

    c Respond with meticulous honesty and fairness in all interactions with clients.

    d Reassure clients that their hallucinations are symptoms of their illness.

20 When the aloof and suspicious client begins to trust the nurse, he or she can be encouraged to participate in which one of the following?

    a Playing Ping-Pong with the nurse.

    b Joining other clients for a card game.

    c Working in the ward dining room.

    d Attending a dance with clients from different wards.

21 When a client expresses delusional ideas, the nurse can be *most* effective by:

    a Pointing out to the client why these ideas are unsound.

    b Explaining away the client's delusions.

    c Listening to the client's beliefs without comment.

    d Encouraging the client to elaborate on the delusions.

22 The nurse initiates a nurse-client relationship with a withdrawn client to:

    a Become a significant other to the client.

    b Implement a variety of interventions within the relationship.

    c Provide unconditional positive feedback to the client.

    d All of the above.

23 Which one of the following human processes is *most* specific to the nursing diagnosis that states: Altered Thought Processes related to delusions (ANA: 2.6.2)?

    a Perception.   c Cognition.

    b Ecological.   d Valuation.

24 Which one of the following nursing actions would be *most* specific to the nursing diagnosis that states: Ineffective Individual Coping related to feelings of helplessness (ANA: 5.5.3, NANDA: 5.1.1.1)?

    a Administering a psychotropic medication to the client.

    b Calling the client by his or her correct name.

    c Limiting the client's decision making.

    d Listening to the client's delusional thinking.

25 When the client's behaviors fail to change after a given period of time, the nurse should do which one of the following *first*?

    a Set more realistic outcome criteria.

    b Identify and work on another nursing goal.

    c Transfer the care of the client to another nurse.

    d Check on the client's current medication dosage.

16 *Individuals with mood disorders*

INTRODUCTION

Whereas schizophrenia is essentially a disorder of thinking reflected in affect and behavior as well as thought, mood disorders are primarily disturbances of affect reflected in thought and action as well as through feelings. Although many people find it difficult to appreciate the schizophrenic response, almost everyone can identify with affective experiences, having felt sadness and depression as well as happiness and joy at some time in their lives. Both depression and joy can occur in varying degrees from mild to severe, from normal to pathologically incapacitating.

Like thought disorders, mood disorders are considered functional, having no demonstrable organic disease associated with them. Also like thought disorders, the cause of mood disorders is not conclusively known. The high incidence of mood disorders among members of the same family, however, suggests that heredity may yet prove to be a significant causative factor. Similarly, biochemical studies have revealed the presence of neuroendocrine abnormalities in individuals suffering from deviations in mood, suggesting a possible physiological cause and/or effect for the development of mood disorders. Other theorists, recognizing the possible influence of emotional and environmental factors, believe that mood disorders may have originated in the developmental years. Unlike schizophrenics, who never experienced a warm and loving relationship in infancy, it is generally believed that persons with a mood disorder experienced a loving, caring, and trusting relationship during infancy. It is hypothesized that sometime in late infancy or early childhood, the individual experienced a cessation of this love. The loss of love at that early time in life may have been real or it may have been fantasized. A real loss, such as of a parent through death or separation, or an imagined or perceived loss, such as might have been the interpretation placed on a parent's shift in attention to a new sibling or the disapproval associated with toilet training, raised a confusing mixture of feelings: love, hate, and anger occurring simultaneously toward the lost love object. Self-doubt and guilt also arise as the individual feels it is wrong to have negative feelings and believes that he or she was somehow responsible for the loss of love. In an effort to regain the lost love the individual repressed and introjected the negative feelings of anger, hate, and guilt and only expressed the warm and loving feelings. In addition, the individual tried to be "good," hardworking, conscientious, and self-sacrificing in an unconscious effort to regain the lost love.

Losses, real or imagined, experienced by the individual later in life evoke feelings reminiscent of the original loss. Some individuals are able to cope with these later losses, emerging stronger and better able to meet life's challenges. Other individuals, however, respond to these losses with feelings of depression, worthlessness, and guilt; loss of interest in life and life's activities; psychomotor agitation or retardation; fatigue and decreased energy; problems eating, sleeping, and communicating; and, often, a preoccupation with death and suicide. Other individuals may respond to a loss with feelings of elation, grandiosity, impulsivity, rapid and excessive speech called flight of ideas, aggressive behaviors, and over-activity. Although these individuals reflect a mood that seems joyful, feelings of anger and hostility are close to the surface and erupt when the individual is thwarted in any way. This characteristic response supports the belief that mania is a defense against underlying depression. Still other individuals respond with a cyclical combination of depressive and manic episodes.

"Mood disorders seriously interfere with the quality of life enjoyed by the affected person and his family. In addition, depression increases the risk of death by suicide. Nurses in all settings have a responsibility to recognize and appro-priately intervene in situations where the individual is experiencing a mood disorder."* The exercises in this chapter are designed to help you review theo-retical concepts basic to an understanding of mood disorders, to apply selected phases of the nursing process to the care of individuals with mood disorders, and to begin to develop some understanding about medications used in the treatment of individuals with a mood disorder.

OBJECTIVES

1. To categorize the various losses experienced in depression.
2. To differentiate between normal grief and depression.
3. To differentiate between the characteristics of the mood disorders, mania and depression.
4. To review therapeutic communication skills used in terminating a nurse-client relationship with a depressed individual.
5. To apply selected phases of the nursing process to clinical situations.
6. To identify the action, dosage, administration, contraindications, precautions, idiosyncrasies, side and adverse effects, and nursing implications relevant to selected medications used in the treatment of clients with mood disorders.

---

*From Taylor CM: Mereness' essentials of psychiatric nursing, ed 13, St Louis, 1990, The CV Mosby Co, chap 16.

1 Psychodynamically, the underlying phenomenon in the development of all mood disorders is loss. Associated with all losses is the loss of self-esteem. Loss can take many forms. The most obvious loss is the loss of a loved one through death, precipitating a depression known as mourning and grief. However, other events can also be perceived as losses and bring on a depressive response. Listed below are fifteen events and eight types of losses. Categorize each event in terms of the loss experienced by checking the boxes in the appropriate columns. Keep in mind that more than one loss may be associated with an event. The first one has been filled in to help you get started.

Event		Losses							
		Self-esteem	Love object	Independence	Freedom	Physical integrity	Youth	Autonomy	Material possessions
1. Laura experienced a severe depression after her first child was born.		☑	☐	☑	☑	☑	☑	☑	☐
2. Vinnie was falsely convicted of a crime, became despondent, and attempted suicide in his cell.		☐	☐	☐	☐	☐	☐	☐	☐
3. Mr. Warren became depressed when he was forced to retire at age 60 because of health problems.		☐	☐	☐	☐	☐	☐	☐	☐
4. Ida became depressed when she broke her leg and was forced to rely on others to get her needs met.		☐	☐	☐	☐	☐	☐	☐	☐
5. Jake has hemophilia and became suicidal when he learned he developed AIDS from contaminated blood transfusions.		☐	☐	☐	☐	☐	☐	☐	☐
6. Blair became despondent and joined the ranks of the homeless after he was fired and evicted from his apartment.		☐	☐	☐	☐	☐	☐	☐	☐
7. Mrs. Ames, a widow, experiences sadness, fatigue, insomnia, and anorexia on the anniversary of her husband's death.		☐	☐	☐	☐	☐	☐	☐	☐
8. When Carol's old dog and faithful companion for many years had to be put to sleep, she became very depressed.		☐	☐	☐	☐	☐	☐	☐	☐
9. After Todd failed his entrance exams and was denied admission to college, he became moody and uncommunicative.		☐	☐	☐	☐	☐	☐	☐	☐
10. Susan has blue spells every year on her birthday.		☐	☐	☐	☐	☐	☐	☐	☐
11. David feels fine as long as he is working but gets restless, irritable, and moody on days off and on vacations.		☐	☐	☐	☐	☐	☐	☐	☐
12. Clint became depressed when his crops were lost in a severe drought.		☐	☐	☐	☐	☐	☐	☐	☐
13. Mark became depressed when his boss and close friend died suddenly and he was promoted to his position.		☐	☐	☐	☐	☐	☐	☐	☐
14. Mrs. Carton's depression developed insidiously when she learned she had cancer and needed radical surgery.		☐	☐	☐	☐	☐	☐	☐	☐
15. Frank became depressed when he lost his home and all its contents to a forest fire raging through his area.		☐	☐	☐	☐	☐	☐	☐	☐

2 List four differences between grief or bereavement and depression.

Grief (bereavement)   *Depression*

a _____   a _____
  _____   _____
  _____   _____

b _____   b _____
  _____   _____
  _____   _____

c _____   c _____
  _____   _____
  _____   _____

d _____   d _____
  _____   _____
  _____   _____

3 Listed below are fifteen characteristics of the mood disorders, mania and/or depression. Differentiate between each one by placing a check in the box or boxes in the appropriate columns. The first one has been filled in to help you get started.

Characteristics	Mood disorders	
	Mania	**Depression**
1. Expressions of guilt	☐	☑
2. Rapid speech, jumping from topic to topic	☐	☐
3. Delusions of grandeur	☐	☐
4. Loss of appetite	☐	☐
5. Agitation	☐	☐
6. Fatigue	☐	☐
7. Psychomotor retardation	☐	☐
8. Sleeplessness	☐	☐
9. Irritability	☐	☐
10. Self-accusatory delusions	☐	☐
11. Feelings of pervasive sadness	☐	☐
12. High energy levels	☐	☐
13. Euphoria	☐	☐
14. Suicidal ideation	☐	☐
15. Elation	☐	☐

4 Read the following situation involving an interaction between a nurse and a client who had been admitted to the hospital following a suicide attempt. Complete the exercises as directed.

  a In the interaction the nurse uses at least ten different therapeutic communication skills to help the client work through her feelings associated with an impending termination of the relationship. Each example of a skill has been italicized and numbered. Place the numbers of the examples in the spaces provided after each communication skill. A communication skill may be illustrated more than once; an example may illustrate more than one skill. The first one has been filled in to help you get started.

Communication Skills

a. Clarifying _____	**f.** Introducing neutral topic _____
b. Encouraging _____	**g.** Making observations ____1____
c. Exploring _____	**h.** Reflecting _____
d. Focusing _____	**i.** Suggesting _____
e. Giving information _____	**j.** Understanding _____

SITUATION: The nurse has developed a nurse-client relationship based on trust. At the onset the nurse identified several nursing objectives, including helping the client to develop a more realistic self-concept, to express her feelings in less self-destructive ways, to relate to others more comfortably, and to plan for her return to the community. However, before all these objectives could be realized, the nurse applied for a leave of absence so that she could return to school. In meeting with Karen the nurse told her client of her plans as the first step in terminating the nurse-client relationship. This is their second interaction since the topic of termination was introduced. After greeting her client by name and waiting for her to respond, the nurse says:

1. **N** *"You are very quiet today."*
   (Pause.)
2. **N** *"Is there anything you would like to talk about?"*
   (Silence.)
3. **N** *"Perhaps we could talk some more about my leaving."*
   C Angrily, "I don't want to talk about it. What good is talking going to do?"
4. **N** *"You sound angry."*
   C "Of course I'm angry. Why shouldn't I be?"
5. **N** *"You feel I am deserting you?"*
   C "Well, aren't you? You're like all the rest."
6. **N** *"All the rest?"*
   (Silence.)
7. **N** *"Go on Karen. Tell me what you are feeling."*
   (Silence.)
8. **N** *"Perhaps it would help to talk about it."*
   C Crying, "I'm sorry. I shouldn't take it out on you. I've brought this on myself."
9. **N** *"I don't understand. What do you mean? How have you brought this on yourself?"*
   C "Getting involved. I should never have let you talk me into working with you."
   (Silence.)

10. **N** *"You have reason to be disappointed and to feel angry. Just when we were getting somewhere, I leave you."*

   C "It's not fair."

11. **N** *"I guess it does seem that way."*
   (Pause.)

12. **N** *"Earlier you said, 'You're like all the rest.' What did you mean by that?"*

   C "I don't know if I can talk about it. It's hard. I don't like to think about it, let alone talk about it. Most of the time I don't, but when you told me you were going away, all the old feelings came rushing back."

13. **N** *"These are painful feelings?"*

   C "I don't like to get involved with anyone. When they go away, I get a panicky feeling."

14. **N** *"Is that what you are feeling now?"*

   C "Yes. I thought it would be different with you, you being a nurse and all. I guess I figured since it was your job, I was safe, that I could always count on you, at least until it was time for me to leave the hospital."

15. **N** *"You thought I would always be there when you needed me and I let you down?"*

   C "Yes. Just like my mother. I counted on her and she went away too."

16. **N** *"What happened?"*
   (Silence.)

   C "When I was a little girl we used to have good times together. She took me to the park and I fed the ducks. She'd buy me a balloon and I'd ride on the merry-go-round. I thought she loved me."

17. **N** *"And then?"*

   C "She killed herself."

18. **N** *"Oh. You've never mentioned this before. I can see this must be difficult for you to talk about."*

   C "It is hard, but it is also a relief to share this with you. Sometimes, even now, I think it must have been my fault. If I had been a better daughter she wouldn't have done it."

19. **N** *"You've been feeling responsible all these years? That's a tough feeling to live with."*

   C "Sometimes it's more than I can bear. I feel so responsible."

20. **N** *"Like before, when you were feeling it was your fault that I'm leaving?"*

   C "I was feeling that if I was a better person you would stay."

21. **N** *"And now? What are you feeling now?"*

   C "Numb. I'm going to miss you. But it isn't my fault, is it? You said you're going back to school? I thought that was just an excuse to get away from me."

22. **N** *"When people feel bad about themselves, it's hard for them not to think everything is their fault."*
   (Silence.)

23. **N** *"It's not your fault. I've always wanted to go back to school to get my degree, and now I have my chance. . . . But I'm going to miss you too and will always remember you."*
   (Pause.)

   C "I feel drained."

24. **N** *"We have been sharing a lot of feelings. That's hard work."*
   (Pause.)

   C "Will we talk some more before you go?"

25. **N** *"Yes, of course. We will continue meeting until the end of the month."*

   C "Tell me again when you start school."

26. **N** *"In about 3 weeks."*
   (Pause.)

27. **N** *"Would you like to talk any more now?"*
    C *"No. I think not. I'm all talked out."*
28. **N** *"Perhaps we have done enough for now."*
29. **N** *"It's 11:45—almost lunch time.*
    (Walking in hall toward dining room.)
30. **N** *"You know, that's something we've never talked about—your favorite foods."*

b Using your understanding of the dynamics of depression, briefly explain why it is essential for Karen to have ample opportunity to work through termination with her nurse.

c Complete the following care plan for Karen. A nursing diagnosis appropriate to termination of the nurse-client relationship has been identified, as well as three nursing objectives. In the space provided give at least one nursing action that the nurse might use with Karen in the remaining 3 weeks to facilitate each of the objectives. Also describe outcome criteria for each of the nursing objectives.

Nursing diagnosis: Anticipatory grieving related to perceived potential loss of significant other (ANA 4.1.1.1, NANDA 9.2.1.2)

Nursing objectives	Nursing actions	Outcome criteria
1. To express feelings associated with the anticipated loss.		
2. To review what has been learned through the relationship.		
3. To transfer positive aspects of the professional relationship to another person or persons.		

5 Listed on p. 141 are six pairs of nursing diagnoses using both the ANA and NANDA diagnostic formats. Each diagnosis reflects a common problem and possible etiological factor for clients exhibiting depression. In the space provided, fill in an appropriate nursing objective and at least two relevant nursing actions for each diagnostic statement. Material for the first diagnosis has been filled in to help you get started.

140

Nursing diagnosis	Objective	Nursing actions
1. Altered Self-Care R/T psychomotor retardation (ANA: 1.3.4) OR Bathing/Hygiene Self-Care Deficit R/T psychomotor retardation (NANDA: 6.5.2).	To help client assume greater responsibility for self-care.	a. Establish and follow a regular hygiene schedule. b. Provide client with soap, towels, etc. c. Stay with client and give direct assistance as needed. d. Allow enough time for the activity and do not rush client.
2. Suicidal Ideation R/T feelings of hopelessness, worthlessness, and despair (ANA: 5.3.2.10) OR Potential for Violence: Self-Directed R/T feelings of hopelessness, worthlessness, and despair (NANDA: 9.2.2).		
3. Psychomotor Retardation R/T feelings of depression and fatigue (ANA: 1.1.2.9) OR Activity Intolerance R/T feelings of depression and fatigue (NANDA: 6.1.1.2).		
4. Refusal to Eat R/T lack of appetite (ANA: 1.3.4.1.5) OR Feeding Self-Care Deficit R/T lack of appetite (NANDA: 6.5.1).		
5. Altered Self-Concept R/T feelings of worthlessness and guilt (ANA: 6.3.2) OR Self-Esteem Disturbance R/T feelings of worthlessness and guilt (NANDA: 7.1.2).		
6. Altered Communication Processes R/T psychomotor retardation (ANA: 5.2.2) OR Impaired Verbal Communication R/T psychomotor retardation (NANDA: 2.1.1.1).		

6 Listed below and on p. 143 are six pairs of nursing diagnoses using both the ANA and NANDA diagnostic formats. Each diagnosis reflects a common problem and possible etiological factor for clients exhibiting manic behaviors. In the space provided, fill in an appropriate nursing objective and at least two relevant nursing actions for each diagnostic statement. Material for the first diagnosis has been filled in to help you get started.

Nursing diagnosis	Objective	Nursing actions
1. Altered Social Interaction R/T unacceptable social behaviors: profane language and sexual aggressiveness (ANA 5.7.2) OR Impaired Social Interaction R/T unacceptable behaviors and profane language (NANDA 3.1.1).	To help client control socially unacceptable behaviors.	a. Accept client. b. Ignore client's profane language. c. Set limits on sexual aggressiveness. d. Distract client with socially acceptable activities, such as Ping-Pong. e. Administer lithium as ordered.
2. Potential Aggression Toward Others R/T elation and poor impulse control (ANA: 5.3.2.5) OR Potential for Violence: Directed at Others R/T elation and poor impulse control (NANDA: 9.2.2).		
3. Altered Self-Care R/T overactivity and an inability to maintain sustained attention (ANA: 1.3.4) OR Dressing/Grooming Self-Care Deficit R/T overactivity and an inability to maintain sustained attention (NANDA: 6.5.3).		

Nursing diagnosis	Objective	Nursing actions
4. Altered Nutrition Processes R/T overactivity (ANA: 7.7.2) OR Altered Nutrition: less than body requirements R/T overactivity (NANDA: 1.1.2.2).		
5. Altered Communication Processes R/T elation and rapid speech pattern (flight of ideas) (ANA: 5.2.2) OR Impaired Verbal Communication R/T elation and rapid speech pattern (flight of ideas) (NANDA: 2.1.1.1).		
6. Potential for Injury R/T poor judgment and impulsivity (ANA: 7.5.1.2) OR Potential for Injury R/T poor judgment and impulsivity (NANDA: 1.6.1).		

7 Individuals with mood disorders are often prescribed one of the mood-elevating drugs or lithium to alleviate their symptoms. Whereas electroconvulsive therapy was commonly used in the past, especially to control depression, it is rarely used now unless clients fail to respond to medications. In this exercise fill in the data on the three drug cards on pp. 144-146. The medications selected are characteristic of the three major types of drugs used in the treatment of mood disorders: tricyclic antidepressants (Desipramine), monoamine oxidase inhibitors (Tranylcypromine), and lithium. Use your psychiatric nursing and pharmacology texts to help you complete the exercise.

(Side one)

Generic name: Desipramine
Trade name(s): Pertofrane, Norpramin

Classification:
Other drugs in this classification:

Action:

Range of daily dosage/route of administration:

Date/client initials/dosage:

Contraindications/precautions:

Drug idiosyncrasies:

(Side two)

Side and adverse effects: Nursing implications for each:

Miscellaneous nursing implications:

Source of data and date:

(Side one)

Generic name: Tranylcypromine
Trade name(s): Parnate

Classification:
Other drugs in this classification:

Action:

Range of daily dosage/route of administration:

Date/client initials/dosage:

Contraindications/precautions:

Drug idiosyncrasies:

(Side two)

Side and adverse effects: Nursing implications for each:

Miscellaneous nursing implications:

Source of data and date:

(Side one)

Generic name: Lithium carbonate
Trade name(s): Eskalith, Lithane

Classification:
Other drugs in this classification:

Action:

Range of daily dosage/route of administration:

Date/client initials/dosage:

Contraindications/precautions:

Drug idiosyncrasies:

(Side two)

Side and adverse effects:	Nursing implications for each:

Miscellaneous nursing implications:

Source of data and date:

TEST ITEMS

DIRECTIONS: Select the *best* response. (Answers appear in the Appendix.)

1 The cyclic nature of mood disorders was first recognized by:
  a Kraepelin.   c Hippocrates.
  b Bleuler.   d Cerletti.

2 Which one of the following behaviors is more characteristic of a person with a thought disorder than a mood disorder?
  a Manifests euphoric mood.
  b Complains of constant fatigue.
  c Exhibits boundless energy.
  d Smiles or laughs inappropriately.

3 Bereavement is a reaction to which one of the following?
  a Real loss of a highly valued object.
  b Symbolic loss of an intangible object.
  c Anticipated loss of a fantasied love object.
  d Imagined loss of a tangible object.

4 One of the phases of normal grief is called:
  a Denial.   c Termination.
  b Restitution.   d Depression.

5 The defense mechanism operating in depression when angry feelings are repressed is *primarily*:
  a Reaction formation.   c Introjection.
  b Rationalization.   d Isolation.

6 The superego in depression is *best* described as:
  a Laissez-faire.   c Punitive.
  b Idealistic.   d Hostile.

7 Which one of the following antidepressants is classified as a monoamine oxidase inhibitor (MAO)?
  a Tofranil (imipramine).   c Sinequan (doxepin).
  b Parnate (tranylcypromine).   d Elavil (amitriptyline).

8 *All but which one* of the following side or adverse effects is common to both MAOs and tricyclics?
  a Dry mouth.   c Hypertensive crisis.
  b Urinary retention.   d Postural hypotension.

9 Which of the following lunch menus would be *most* appropriate for a person taking Marplan (isocarboxazid)?
  a Grilled cheese sandwich, apple pie, black coffee.
  b Spaghetti and meatballs, chocolate pudding, milk.
  c Hamburger on a bun, french fries, diet soda.
  d Chopped chicken liver on rye bread, tossed salad, tea.

10 Lithium toxicity can *best* be prevented by monitoring which one of the following?
   a Urine for excretion of the drug.
   b Blood for elevated white count.
   c Blood pressure for signs of hypertension.
   d Serum for drug levels.

11 Symptoms of lithium toxicity include which one of the following?
   a Ocular changes.
   b Abdominal cramps.
   c Pseudoparkinsonism.
   d Confusion.

12 The hyperactive client is receiving lithium carbonate daily. Which one of the following nursing measures is *most* indicated?
   a Arranging a regular schedule of blood work.
   b Checking vital signs four times a day (q.i.d.).
   c Limiting fluid intake to 1000 ml per day.
   d Taking the blood pressure before administering medication.

13 One of the common temporary side effects of electroconvulsive therapy occurring after five or six treatments is:
   a Postural hypotension.
   b Urinary incontinence.
   c Muscle weakness.
   d Loss of memory.

14 Which one of the following symptoms is *most* associated with psychomotor retardation?
   a Severe anxiety.
   b Feelings of worthlessness.
   c Marked agitation.
   d Constant fatigue.

15 Which one of the following human processes is *most* specific to the nursing diagnosis that states: Altered Home Maintenance R/T fatigue and inactivity (ANA: 3.3.2)?
   a Ecological.
   b Cognition.
   c Emotional.
   d Valuation.

16 Which one of the following is a fallacy about suicide?
   a People who talk about suicide are thinking about suicide.
   b Introducing the topic of suicide to a depressed person will precipitate a suicide attempt.
   c Suicide attempts are usually preceded by some warning.
   d Almost every person who makes a suicide attempt is suffering from depression.

17 Depressed clients are prone to physical disorders such as constipation primarily because of their:
   a Preoccupation with their bodily functions.
   b Inactivity and lack of physical exercise.
   c Failure to seek prompt medical help for their health problems.
   d All of the above.

18 Which one of the following nursing approaches would be *most* helpful and realistic to use with a very depressed person?

a Presenting a cheerful, energetic manner to clients.

b Expecting clients to take initiative in self-care.

c Providing clients with opportunities for decision making.

d Establishing a simple daily schedule of activities for clients.

19 Which one of the following nursing responses would be *most* specific to the nursing diagnosis that states: Activity Intolerance R/T psychomotor retardation (NANDA: 6.1.1.2)?

a Consistency.   b Firmness.   c Patience.   d Honesty.

20 The purpose of assigning menial tasks such as cleaning the bathroom to depressed clients is to provide them with tasks that:

a Relieve their feelings of guilt.

b Distract them from their unhappy thoughts.

c Raise their self-esteem.

d Reduce their tension and fatigue.

21 The *most* effective nursing measure to protect the depressed client from self-destructive tendencies is to:

a Remove all potentially lethal weapons from the environment.

b Provide close supervision by staying with the client.

c Administer the maximum dosage of antidepressants during acute periods.

d Place the client in seclusion in a barren room.

22 Which one of the following objectives is applicable to *all* acutely ill elated and hyperactive clients?

a Control their use of loud and vulgar language.

b Protect them and others from their impulsive behavior.

c Maintain their contacts with the members of their family.

d Protect them from their unconscious suicidal impulses.

23 Listed below are four menus. Which one would be *both* nutritious and appropriate to serve to a hyperactive individual?

a Spaghetti and meatballs, salad, banana.

b Beef and vegetable stew, bread, vanilla pudding.

c Broiled chicken leg, ear of corn, apple.

d Fried fish sticks, stewed tomatoes, chocolate cake.

24 Which one of the following activities would be the *least* appropriate outlet for the manic individual's excess energy?

a Team sports.   b Folding linen.   c Writing.   d Drawing.

25 In response to the overactive, elated individual's vulgar speech and seductive behavior, the nurse can be *most* helpful by:

a Responding to the client with understanding and acceptance.

b Pointing out to the client that the behaviors are bad.

c Telling the client he or she will be punished if he or she does not behave.

d Avoiding the client until he or she can control the behavior.

17 | *Individuals with anxiety disorders*

INTRODUCTION

Anxiety is an energy force that promotes activity and productivity on the one hand and interferes with functioning on the other. In thought disorders, anxiety restricts logical thinking, reality perception, and relatedness with others. In mood disorders, anxiety seems to propel individuals into flurries of disorganized activity or to reduce them to energyless states of depression. Individuals with both thought and mood disorders are all psychotic. In anxiety disorders nonpsychotic individuals attempt to control high levels of anxiety through the use of characteristic behavioral patterns: repetitive rituals (obsessive-compulsive disorders), physical symptoms with no organic basis (conversion disorders), unrealistic and generally unfounded fears (phobic disorders), and disturbances in identity, memory, and/ or consciousness (multiple personality disorder).

Prior to 1980 and the revised classification of psychiatric disorders, individuals experiencing these behavioral patterns were labeled neurotic. According to Freud individuals suffering from a neurosis (psychoneurosis) were experiencing extreme anxiety arising out of intrapsychic conflicts, conflicts among the id, ego, and superego. He believed these individuals to be nonpsychotic, in touch with reality, and suitable candidates for treatment with psychoanalysis. Some current theorists believe that psychotic individuals also experience intrapsychic conflicts and can benefit from some forms of psychotherapy. The use of the term *neurosis* became controversial, and, in an effort to acknowledge the current thinking, it was discarded and the less controversial and more descriptive phrase *anxiety disorder* was adopted. However, despite the change in terminology, the theoretical understanding of these disorders still reflects a markedly Freudian interpretation. Little if any significant research in the fields of genetics or biochemistry has suggested new factors contributing to the cause of these disorders. Emotional factors are still largely identified as the predisposing factors contributing to the development of the Anxiety Disorders.

150

Individuals with anxiety disorders differ from persons with thought and mood disorders in that they have a greater degree of ego strength. This is reflected in behavior. They are in touch with reality and possess varying degrees of insight that they are not experiencing life to its fullest. Their relationships with others may become strained, but, despite this, they rarely withdraw but instead reach out to others for help. Although they utilize repression, in combination with other ego defenses, to keep unconscious conflicts out of awareness, they can engage in problem solving with some success and are generally able to take action to seek help and relief from their increasingly incapacitating symptoms. Their memory is usually intact and their judgment fairly sound, except when anxiety reaches extreme proportions.

"Because individuals suffering from anxiety disorders are in touch with reality and often recognize the inappropriateness of their behavior, many nurses have difficulty accepting them as persons in need of health care. To achieve a more understanding attitude toward these individuals, it is important to develop some knowledge about the emotional conflicts with which they struggle and the ways in which they use symptoms to cope with the anxiety that stems from these conflicts."* The exercises in this chapter are designed to help you develop a greater understanding of individuals with anxiety disorders, to apply selected phases of the nursing process to their care, and to begin to develop some understanding about the use of anxiolytic medications in the treatment of individuals with an anxiety disorder.

OBJECTIVES

1. To review theoretical concepts basic to an understanding of individuals with anxiety disorders.
2. To apply selected phases of the nursing process to clinical situations.
3. To identify the action, dosage, administration, contraindications, precautions, idiosyncrasies, side and adverse effects, and nursing implications relevant to the use of anxiolytic medications.

---

*From Taylor CM: Mereness' essentials of psychiatric nursing, ed 13, St Louis, 1990, The CV Mosby Co, chap 17.

1 According to Freudian theory all anxiety disorders arise out of unresolved conflicts originating in one or more of the pregenital stages of psychosexual development, namely, the oral, anal, and/or phallic stages. For example, a continued conflict with cleanliness first experienced in the anal stage can predispose an individual to the development of an obsessive-compulsive disorder as manifested by a preoccupation with cleanliness and compulsive, ritualistic behaviors aimed at keeping clean and neat. Listed below are fifteen experiences that normally characterize the pregenital stages but that, if unresolved at the time, may create intrapsychic conflict and contribute to the development of an anxiety disorder later in life. Read each one and place a check in the box in the appropriate column. The first experience has been filled in to help you get started.

Pregenital experiences	Stages of development		
	Oral	Anal	Phallic
The individual:			
1. Experiences an expectation to be clean.	☐	☑	☐
2. Feels narcissistic.	☐	☐	☐
3. Engages in masturbation.	☐	☐	☐
4. Experiences toilet training.	☐	☐	☐
5. Seeks instant gratification with the mouth.	☐	☐	☐
6. Experiences weaning.	☐	☐	☐
7. Feels omnipotent.	☐	☐	☐
8. Associates pleasure with bowel/bladder evacuation.	☐	☐	☐
9. Experiences incestuous feelings toward opposite-sex parent.	☐	☐	☐
10. Learns to postpone pleasure.	☐	☐	☐
11. Associates food and eating with love.	☐	☐	☐
12. Experiences penis envy/castration fears.	☐	☐	☐
13. Is helpless and entirely dependent on others.	☐	☐	☐
14. Experiences tension in penis/clitoris.	☐	☐	☐
15. Engages in sibling rivalry.	☐	☐	☐

2 The three parts of the personality—the id, ego, and superego—all play a role in the development and/or resolution of intrapsychic conflicts that may contribute to the development of anxiety disorders.

a Listed below are twenty characteristics of the id, the ego, or the superego. Read each one and place a check in the box in the appropriate column. The first one has been filled in to help you get started.

Characteristics	Parts of the personality		
	Id	Ego	Superego
1. Innate, ruthless, primitive, and selfish.	☑	☐	☐
2. Operates on basis of pleasure-pain principle.	☐	☐	☐
3. Develops out of socialization process.	☐	☐	☐
4. Strict, rigid, and moralistic.	☐	☐	☐
5. Engages in reality testing.	☐	☐	☐
6. Seeks immediate gratification.	☐	☐	☐
7. Rational and reasonable.	☐	☐	☐
8. Represents the self to others.	☐	☐	☐
9. Source of all libidinal pleasure.	☐	☐	☐
10. Contains drives for self-preservation.	☐	☐	☐
11. Punishes by invoking anxiety and guilt.	☐	☐	☐
12. Incorporates ideals learned from others.	☐	☐	☐
13. Consists of conscience and ego ideal.	☐	☐	☐
14. Develops out of interaction with the environment.	☐	☐	☐
15. Effects compromises.	☐	☐	☐
16. Rewards desirable behavior.	☐	☐	☐
17. Utilizes defense mechanisms to control anxiety.	☐	☐	☐
18. Operates on basis of reality principle.	☐	☐	☐
19. Conscious part of personality.	☐	☐	☐
20. Incorporates taboos learned from others.	☐	☐	☐

b In the space provided briefly describe the role of the id, ego, and superego in the development or resolution of intrapsychic conflicts that may contribute to the development of an anxiety disorder.

3 The use of defenses in characteristic patterns reflects the nature of anxiety disorders, somatoform disorders, and dissociative disorders. For example, in the anxiety disorders of phobic and obsessive-compulsive disorders, the mechanisms utilized are displacement, preoccupation, and symbolism. In phobias the preoccupation is with the object of fear that is avoided to control anxiety; in compulsions the preoccupation, or obsession, is a thought that keeps recurring. By focusing on one thought the individual is able to avoid focusing on thoughts that would be more troubling and anxiety producing. In addition, undoing is operating when the individual compulsively carries out repetitive acts to try to blot out the troubling thought as well as magically erase or "undo" the unconscious conflict, anxiety, and guilt that underlie these behaviors. In the somatoform disorders of conversion disorder, the defenses of conversion and symbolism are used consistently. In fact, the use of conversion is exclusive to this disorder. In dissociative disorders, such as multiple personality disorder, the mechanism of dissociation is used, whereby certain aspects of the personality escape from the individual's control, become separated from consciousness, and function as a separate identity. Finally, all these disorders utilize the defense mechanism of repression, trying to keep the unconscious conflicts out of awareness.

Listed below and on p. 155 are twelve examples of behaviors associated with selected defenses. Read each one and identify which defenses are operating by placing a check in the box in the appropriate column. The first one has been filled in to help you get started.

	Defenses						
Behavioral responses	Displacement	Symbolism	Conversion	Preoccupation	Undoing	Repression	Dissociation
1. Edwardo was obsessed with the belief that he was dying of a brain tumor, although multiple physical examinations and laboratory tests did not support his fears.	☑	☑	☐	☑	☑	☑	☐
2. Roger's father, a military man, hoped that his son would also follow a military career. After graduation from high school Roger enlisted in the infantry but was unable to report for duty because of sudden, unexplained paralysis in his legs. No organic reason could be found for his symptoms.	☐	☐	☐	☐	☐	☐	☐

Behavioral responses	Defenses						
	Displacement	Symbolism	Conversion	Preoccupation	Undoing	Repression	Dissociation
3. One day Mike was mistakenly locked in a closet for 10 hours while playing in an abandoned building. He was 7 years old. As an adult he had no recall of the incident but continued to experience severe anxiety when alone in windowless areas such as elevators, closets, or enclosed stairwells.	☐	☐	☐	☐	☐	☐	☐
4. Helen's freedom of movement was severely restricted because of recurring thoughts that she had neglected to turn off the water in the sink before leaving the house. She acknowledged that her fears were groundless, but she could not resist the urge to return home to check out her concerns.	☐	☐	☐	☐	☐	☐	☐
5. When Thelma was 6 years old she was physically threatened by her mother for masturbating. Thelma never masturbated again and never mentioned the incident to anyone. Years later when she engaged in heavy petting with a boyfriend, she experienced a severe anxiety attack. The next day she awoke with an unexplained paralysis of both hands. She felt little concern over the incapacitating symptoms.	☐	☐	☐	☐	☐	☐	☐
6. Melissa was sexually abused by her father when she was a child. Years later, in psychotherapy, it was revealed she had twelve different identities.	☐	☐	☐	☐	☐	☐	☐
7. Watson became panicky when faced with air travel. This had not been a problem until his job required extensive travel. For days before a trip Watson could think about nothing else. In therapy he revealed that his father had died in a plane crash when he was 6 years old and he had felt guilty about it for years.	☐	☐	☐	☐	☐	☐	☐
8. Everything about Katie was meticulous: her appearance, her home, and her work. Every night after work she carried out elaborate cleaning procedures before eating dinner. She would take the telephone off the hook so she would not be disturbed. Any interference caused her great stress, and she was forced to start her ritual over from the beginning.	☐	☐	☐	☐	☐	☐	☐
9. Fran had a morbid fear of the dark. This was a childhood fear and she had apparently "outgrown" it. However, shortly after she married, the old thoughts recurred, and she insisted that all the lights be left on in the apartment. The marriage was now in peril because she would not sleep without a bright light in the bedroom and her husband had moved out into the living room.	☐	☐	☐	☐	☐	☐	☐
10. Lucy still lived at home with her parents. It was a close-knit but undemonstrative family. She rarely was kissed by her parents and had never seen them embrace. One day she came home from work early and found her parents in the act of sexual intercourse. She experienced a confusing mixture of horror and sexual stimulation. The next morning she awakened and could not see.	☐	☐	☐	☐	☐	☐	☐
11. Tina was very concerned with her weight. She weighed and measured all her food before eating it, after making meticulous calculations of caloric values. She also weighed herself before and after every meal and kept elaborate records of her intake. Any distractions that interfered with her completing her rituals caused Tina great anxiety.	☐	☐	☐	☐	☐	☐	☐
12. Jenny's friends could not understand her strange behavior. She assumed the identity of multiple personalities, each of which had different names and distinctive behavioral patterns.	☐	☐	☐	☐	☐	☐	☐

4 Listed below are the eight human processes under which symptomatology may be organized according to the ANA Classification of Human Responses of Concern for Psychiatric–Mental Health Nursing Practice, Draft IV-R (September 20, 1988). In the space provided describe at least one behavior specific to each one of the processes that is characteristically exhibited by individuals experiencing anxiety disorders. Material for the first one has been filled in to help you get started.

   a Activity Processes: restlessness (pacing), repetitive behaviors (rituals), failure to carry out self-care, sleeplessness.

   b Cognition Processes:

   c Ecological Processes:

   d Emotional Processes:

   e Interpersonal Processes:

   f Perception Processes:

   g Physiological Processes:

   h Valuation Processes:

5 Read each of the following mini-situations involving individuals experiencing symptoms of Anxiety Disorders. In the space provided, write a *pair* of nursing diagnoses using both the ANA and NANDA diagnostic formats, *one* nursing objective, and at least *two* nursing actions appropriate to each identified problem. Material for the first mini-situation has been filled in to help you get started.

a MINI-SITUATION: Ellen George, a housewife, is so anxious that she is unable to complete any household tasks she starts. The fact that her home is untidy and unclean adds to her anxiety.

Nursing diagnoses	Nursing objective	Nursing actions
Altered Home Maintenance R/T anxiety stemming from unconscious conflicts (ANA: 3.3.2) AND Impaired Home Maintenance R/T anxiety stemming from unconscious conflicts (NANDA: 6.4.1.1).	To help decrease client's anxiety.	1. Administer anxiolytic medications as ordered. 2. Work with family to temporarily relieve client of most home maintenance activities. 3. Encourage client to identify and carry out short-term projects such as scrub the sink rather than clean the entire kitchen. 4. Listen with an accepting attitude to the client's concerns and feelings. 5. Tell client about the availability of different types of therapy.

b MINI-SITUATION: Martha Roy has such extreme anxiety that she is unable to concentrate on any activity for very long. She paces the floor for hours and chain-smokes.

Nursing diagnoses	Nursing objective	Nursing actions

c MINI-SITUATION: Jerome Jackson conducts a very profitable mail order business out of his home. However, multiple fears interfere with his social life as he refuses to go outdoors.

Nursing diagnoses	Nursing objective	Nursing actions

d MINI-SITUATION: Laura Morgan sought professional help and was diagnosed as having multiple personality disorder. She is very ambivalent about being in therapy. She believes that it is a sign of weakness and that she should be able to control her problems herself.

Nursing diagnoses	Nursing objective	Nursing actions

e MINI-SITUATION: Suzanne Lloyd, a secretary, is having increasing difficulties functioning at work because of her preoccupation with order. Before beginning any task she must first line up all her pens, pencils, and paper clips in a precise order. If interrupted, she becomes anxious and must begin again.

Nursing diagnoses	Nursing objective	Nursing actions

f MINI-SITUATION: Sarah Grant is obsessed with her body and its functioning. She frequently visits different physicians with complaints of dizziness, shortness of breath, loss of appetite, diarrhea, palpitations, and sensations of tightness in her stomach, head, and throat.

Nursing diagnoses	Nursing objective	Nursing actions

6 In addition to relieving anxiety in nonpsychotic individuals, anxiolytic medications may be used to control other problems. In the space provided list three other uses for these medications.

a _____

b _____

c _____

7 Select one of the anxiolytic medications and fill in the data on the following drug card.

(Side one)

Generic name:
Trade name:
Classification:
Other drugs in this classification:
Action:
Range of daily dosage/route of administration:
Date/client initials/dosage:
Contraindications/precautions:
Drug idiosyncrasies:

(Side two)

| Side and adverse effects: | Nursing implications for each: |

Miscellaneous nursing implications:

Source of data and date:

TEST ITEMS

DIRECTIONS: Select the *best* response. (Answers appear in the Appendix.)

1 Anxiety disorders include *all but which one* of the following?
   a Conversion disorder.   c Simple phobia.
   b Obsessive-compulsive disorder.   d Panic disorder.

2 A person with a social phobia would be *most* fearful of which one of the following?
   a Enclosed areas.   c Group situations.
   b Specific animals.   d High places.

3 Another term for obsession is:
   a Compulsion.   c Preoccupation.
   b Ritual.   d Fear.

4 Post-traumatic disorders are characterized by which one of the following?
   a Fear of flying.
   b Physical symptoms.
   c Splitting off of the personality.
   d Flashbacks of terrifying experiences.

5 Persons with conversion disorders manifest which one of the following?
   a Indifference to their symptoms.   c Multiple physical problems.
   b Anger at being incapacitated.   d Extreme anxiety.

6 Persons suffering from multiple personality disorder are usually found to have experienced which one of the following in their childhood years?

 a Sibling rivalry.   c Oedipal/Electra conflict.

 b Sexual assault.   d Parental abandonment.

7 According to intrapsychic theory the symptoms associated with anxiety disorders develop:

 a When repression fails to keep troublesome conflicts out of consciousness.

 b As a dysfunctional adaptation to anxiety and stress.

 c In an effort to bring relief from conflicts associated with primitive impulses.

 d All of the above.

8 The use of anxiolytic medications is generally contraindicated in the treatment of crisis states because they tend to do which of the following?

 a Promote long-term physical dependency.

 b Mask the symptoms of underlying depression.

 c Decrease the motivation to face problems.

 d Interfere with mental acuity.

9 In addition to reducing anxiety, anxiolytic medications are used to do which of the following?

 a Potentiate anticonvulsant medications.

 b Relieve muscle spasm.

 c Treat alcohol withdrawal.

 d All of the above.

10 If a client on an anxiolytic medication develops a paradoxical response, the nurse should immediately notify the physician and:

 a Withhold the medication.

 b Administer an antiallergic medication as ordered.

 c Put the client to bed in a darkened room.

 d Carry out dietary restrictions.

11 The *most* effective long-term treatments of anxiety disorders are:

 a Behavior modification.   c Desensitization.

 b Anxiolytic medications.   d Psychotherapy.

12 Supportive psychotherapy is to coping with problems as insight psychotherapy is to:

 a Uncovering unconscious material.

 b Dealing with current stressors.

 c Reducing extremes of anxiety.

 d Repressing painful experiences.

13 The individual who is the *most* suitable candidate for insight psychotherapy is one who:

 a Appears to have a strong ego.

 b Lacks resources and needs support.

 c Has a long-term psychotic illness.

 d Needs help in verbalizing problems.

14 Which one of the following nursing diagnoses would be *most* specific to clients with an obsessive-compulsive disorder?
    a Altered Sleep/Arousal Patterns R/T high anxiety (ANA: 1.4.2).
    b Altered Motor Behavior R/T chronic fatigue (ANA: 1.1.2).
    c Altered Social Interaction R/T fear of speaking in public (ANA: 5.7.2).
    d Altered Home Maintenance R/T preoccupation with dirt (ANA: 3.3.2).

15 Nursing objectives appropriate to the care of *all* individuals with anxiety disorders are to reduce anxiety and:
    a Face reality that underlying conflicts cannot be treated.
    b Develop alternate adaptations to anxiety-producing situations.
    c Strive for insight into intrapsychic conflicts.
    d Learn to control primitive sexual impulses.

16 The person who must control anxiety with elaborate repetitive rituals will experience the greatest security if the nurse does which one of the following?
    a Distracts him with other activities.
    b Encourages him to talk about the purpose of his rituals.
    c Allows him to carry out his rituals.
    d Limits the time he spends in ritualistic activities.

17 Jason is admitted to a surgical service for hernia repair. On the admission interview he tells the nurse that he is morbidly afraid of the dark. Which one of the following responses by the nurse would be the *most* helpful to the client?
    a "How long have you been afraid of the dark?"
    b "Would you feel more comfortable if a light is kept on in your room?"
    c "Afraid of the dark? It's OK. You don't need to be afraid here."
    d "That must be very inconvenient sometimes."

18 Encouraging anxious clients to participate in recreational and/or occupational activities serves *all but which one* of the following purposes?
    a Develop new interests.   c Release physical tension.
    b Promote group interactions.   d Provide emotional insights.

19 Short-term hospitalization is generally indicated for anxious clients to provide them with which one of the following?
    a Neutral environment.   c Stimulating challenges.
    b Decision-making opportunities.   d Physical care.

20 In initiating a conversation with the anxious client the nurse might *most* appropriately begin by:
    a Asking how the client feels.
    b Focusing on a neutral topic of mutual interest.
    c Giving the client a choice of an activity in which to join.
    d All of the above.

18

Individuals with psychophysiological disorders

INTRODUCTION

"The phenomenon referred to as *somatization* is a process whereby an individual's feelings, emotional needs, or conflicts are manifested physiologically. When the need, feeling, or conflict is on a conscious level the somatization process occurs as an adaptation to the stress of the emotion. When the emotion is on an unconscious level, somatization also serves the function of defending the individual against conscious awareness of the nature of the emotion. In either instance the process of somatization supports the widely accepted belief that the functions and reactions of the mind and body are inextricably related." *

It can be safely stated that everyone has at some time been affected with physical symptoms in response to emotional experiences. Pallor and perspiration in response to fear, blushing and stuttering induced by embarrassment, headaches and muscle stiffness brought on by tension, nausea and vomiting precipitated by anxiety, palpitations and insomnia evoked by nervous anticipation, and vegetative symptoms such as constipation and anorexia associated with depression are all examples of symptomatic expressions demonstrating the close relationship between the mind (and emotions) and the body. In some instances the physiological response heightens awareness of the emotional experience. Such is the situation with love, pleasurable anticipation, and mild anxiety. The response can be stimulating and at times exciting. In other instances, such as with increasing fear and anxiety, the physiological response serves to mobilize the individual into action, to take flight or perhaps to stand and fight in a threatening situation. In cases in which the physical symptoms are observable to others, they serve as modes of nonverbal communication to the astute observer.

---

*From Taylor CM: Mereness' essentials of psychiatric nursing, ed 13, St Louis, 1990, The CV Mosby Co, chap 18.

If these somatic responses to emotional situations are sustained and produce measurable changes in the body's organs, the individual is said to have a psychophysiological disorder. Although there is still some resistance to the belief that the functions and reactions of the mind and body are closely intertwined, most people acknowledge that a few disorders may have such a relationship. Peptic ulcers, bronchial asthma, and eczema fall into this category. The belief that a relationship exists between the physical symptoms of other conditions such as essential hypertension, ulcerative colitis, and rheumatoid arthritis and the underlying emotional factors contributing to their onset still evokes disbelief. The idea that a mind-body relationship exists with still other conditions such as tuberculosis, coronary heart disease, and cancer is met with outspoken skepticism. Despite these different responses, there is growing evidence to support the belief that *all* physical illnesses are inextricably bound up with an individual's emotional state and personality structure.

The exercises in this chapter are designed to help you heighten your awareness of the role emotions play in everyday life, to increase your understanding of psychophysiological disorders, and to apply selected phases of the nursing process to the care of individuals with these disorders.

OBJECTIVES

1. To identify the emotional component in everyday figures of speech related to parts of the body.
2. To differentiate among somatization, conversion, hypochondriasis, and malingering.
3. To differentiate between primary and secondary gains of an illness.
4. To describe nursing actions that discourage secondary gains and somatization.
5. To apply selected phases of the nursing process to clinical situations.

1 The relationship between mind and body is often expressed in everyday conversation. The English language is filled with idiomatic expressions that use a part of the body to symbolically reflect emotions. The expression "She turned a deaf ear to his plea" is an example of "body language" in which indifference is clearly being expressed. The following list of fifteen idioms is a sampling of emotions expressed verbally through reference to a body part. Read each one and in the adjoining space identify the feeling message that is being communicated. The first one has been filled in to help you get started. Additional space is provided for you to enter other "body language" idiomatic expressions that you may use to communicate your feelings.

Idiomatic expression	Feeling message
1. "My stomach was in my throat."	Fear, anxiety
2. "He's got a heart of stone."	
3. "She makes my skin crawl."	
4. "He was up in arms when he heard the news."	
5. "Keep a stiff upper lip."	
6. "He's too thick-skinned."	
7. "She tried to save face by lying."	
8. "That turns my stomach."	
9. "He fell head over heels with her."	
10. "You give me a pain in the butt."	
11. "He's a hard-nosed individual."	
12. "You're a sight for sore eyes."	
13. "She gave him the cold shoulder."	
14. "I'm all ears."	
15. "My hair stood on end."	
16.	
17.	
18.	
19.	
20.	

2 Four phenomena are often confused: somatization, conversion, hypochondriasis, and malingering. Somatization is a process by which anxiety is expressed through physical symptoms that have an organic basis and in which physiological changes can be demonstrated in the involved organ. Conversion is a process by which anxiety is controlled through physical symptoms that have no organic basis and in which there is no demonstrable change in the body part. Hypochondriasis is a state of mind in which the individual experiences a heightened awareness of, and preoccupation with, bodily functions despite the fact that there are no demonstrable physical symptoms or physiological changes in the organs involved. Malingering is a purposeful, conscious feigning or faking of illness or injury in the absence of any physical problem in order to derive secondary gains, such as monetary rewards. In the following exercise read each of the fifteen behavioral manifestations listed and differentiate among somatization, conversion, hypochondriasis, and malingering by placing a check in the box in the appropriate column. The first one has been filled in to help you get started.

Behavioral manifestations	Somatization	Conversion	Hypochondriasis	Malingering
1. Morgan lied about having the flu so he could stay home to watch the World Series.	☐	☐	☐	☑
2. Linda experiences severe migraine headaches when under stress.	☐	☐	☐	☐
3. Hannah goes from one physician to another seeking reassurance that she does not have cancer even though no pathology has been identified.	☐	☐	☐	☐
4. Jack pretended to have symptoms of whiplash following a car accident in hopes of collecting disability insurance.	☐	☐	☐	☐
5. Barbara developed an unexplained paralysis of her right hand after she beat her son.	☐	☐	☐	☐
6. Marco's stomach ulcer flares up before he has to lecture, and he takes antacids for temporary relief.	☐	☐	☐	☐
7. Flora's mother died from cardiovascular disease. Since then Flora has been obsessed with her heart and blood pressure and bought a blood pressure apparatus to check her blood pressure six or seven times a day.	☐	☐	☐	☐
8. Dale is allergic to dogs and develops upper respiratory–like symptoms when in close contact with them.	☐	☐	☐	☐
9. Lena developed sudden and unexplained blindness after witnessing her parents making love.	☐	☐	☐	☐

Continued.

167

Behavioral manifestations	Somatization	Conversion	Hypochondriasis	Malingering
10. Tim faked physical symptoms to avoid an undesirable work assignment.	☐	☐	☐	☐
11. Tom joined the police department to please his father but developed an unexplained paralysis of his "trigger finger" when he began handling firearms.	☐	☐	☐	☐
12. Laura is very focused on her health and bodily functions and takes twenty-five vitamins and mineral tablets a day. She also has frequent physical check-ups with different doctors.	☐	☐	☐	☐
13. Myra awakened on her wedding day to find she was paralyzed and could not walk. Examinations and lab tests failed to reveal an organic reason for the paralysis.	☐	☐	☐	☐
14. Jeanne was very close to her mother, and when the mother died Jeanne developed severe asthma.	☐	☐	☐	☐
15. Cliff told his mother he felt sick to his stomach to avoid going to school where he was scheduled to take an important test.	☐	☐	☐	☐

3 The individual with a psychophysiological disorder generally has no insight into why a particular symptom develops or what purpose it serves. The fact that an unconscious conflict is being kept out of awareness by the combined use of repression and somatization is unknown to the client. What is experienced is the control of anxiety. This relief from anxiety is the purpose of developing the symptoms and is called the *primary gain* of the illness. In addition to the primary gain, the client on occasion may experience a *secondary gain* from the illness. Secondary gains occur when the client experiences attention, sympathy, material benefits, special consideration, and control over others and, in effect, seems to be rewarded for being ill. Although some secondary gains are to be expected and perhaps are even desirable, the nurse needs to be aware that they can prolong an illness by unconsciously reinforcing the pattern of somatization. An understanding that primary gains control anxiety is the theoretical basis for allowing a client to retain his patterns of behavior and to relinquish them at his own pace. Similarly, an understanding that a client may consciously or unconsciously retain these same patterns of behavior because of their secondary gains is the theoretical basis for using nursing activities that do not unduly reinforce these gains and interfere with the client's recovery.

a Listed below are ten behavioral examples that reflect either primary (I°) or secondary (II°) gains. Differentiate between each one by placing a check in the box in the appropriate column. The first one has been filled in to help you get started.

	Gains	
Behavioral examples	**I°**	**II°**
1. Carl did not mind staying home when he was sick because he could watch baseball games on TV.	☐	☑
2. Mookie's peptic ulcer is a somatic expression of an unconscious emotional conflict.	☐	☐
3. Harry collected disability insurance after he injured his hand on the assembly line at work.	☐	☐
4. Susan anticipates having her mother make her favorite chicken soup whenever she is ill.	☐	☐
5. Mary, disabled with rheumatoid arthritis, appears kind and self-sacrificing and is unaware of her repressed feelings of anger and rage.	☐	☐
6. Mark's unconscious need to conform to the expectations of others is expressed in an elevated blood pressure.	☐	☐
7. Sue's chronic asthma reflects her unconscious ambivalent feelings toward her mother.	☐	☐
8. Jose looked forward to receiving cards and telephone calls from his friends while he was recuperating.	☐	☐
9. Jennifer developed skin rashes when facing stressful events in her life.	☐	☐
10. Webster's friends rallied to his side when they learned he was terminally ill.	☐	☐

b List three nursing actions that could be taken to avoid reinforcing secondary gains.

1. _____

_____

2. _____

_____

3. _____

_____

4 In the assessment phase of the nursing process the nurse collects, validates, and analyzes data. In the following exercise describe the physical and emotional factors contributing to the onset of symptoms in individuals with psychophysiological disorders. The first one has been filled in to help you get started.

Psychophysiologic disorders	Physical factors	Emotional factors
1. Ulcerative colitis	Gastrointestinal disorder in which the blood supply to the bowel is reduced, leading to ischemia and the formation of ulcers in the walls of the bowel.	Prior to the onset of symptoms the individual experiences ambivalent feelings toward the mother and conflict over dependency needs. Obsessive-compulsive features are used to control others. Anger and rage are internalized and expressed symbolically through physical symptoms.
2. Peptic ulcer		
3. Essential hypertension		
4. Bronchial asthma		
5. Rheumatoid arthritis		

5 A major principle of psychiatric nursing that has particular relevance in caring for individuals with psychophysiologic disorders is the "holistic principle." This principle states that the nurse views the client as a holistic being with a multiplicity of interrelated and interdependent needs. Read each one of the following mini-situations involving individuals experiencing a psychophysiologic disorder. In the space provided write *one* nursing diagnosis for each client, identify at least *two* nursing objectives, and list at least *two* nursing actions appropriate to each objective. Use the ANA Classification of Human Responses of Concern for Psychiatric–Mental Health Nursing Practice.* Each diagnostic statement should reflect use of the holistic principle and an understanding of the mind-body relationship that exists in each disorder. One nursing objective should focus on the client's physical problem, and one should focus on the client's emotional needs. Material for the first one has been filled in to help you get started.

    a MINI-SITUATION: Emma Reynolds, a computer programmer, was admitted to the medical service for treatment of chronic ulcerative colitis. She was experiencing severe abdominal cramps, anorexia, nausea and vomiting, and general malaise. She evacuated as many as 12 to 15 loose, foul-smelling stools daily, containing blood, mucous, and pus. She was very anxious and expressed concern about her symptoms.

Nursing diagnosis	Nursing objectives	Nursing actions
Altered Elimination Process R/T unconscious feelings of ambivalence and repressed rage (ANA: 7.2.2).	Physical: Help restore client's physiological homeokinesis.	1. Provide bed rest. 2. Give skin care. 3. Observe and record the number and nature of daily stools. 4. Provide ventilation, air fresheners. 5. Give balanced diet, fluids. 6. Administer medications as ordered.
	Emotional: Help reduce client's anxiety.	7. Anticipate needs. 8. Listen to client's concerns. 9. Tell client about psychotherapy.

*See Taylor CM: Mereness' essentials of psychiatric nursing, ed 13, St Louis, 1990, The CV Mosby Co, Appendix E, for help with this exercise.

b MINI-SITUATION: Franklyn Keck, an advertising executive, was admitted to the medical service for a work-up for a possible peptic ulcer. On admission he complained of gnawing, aching, burning pain in his upper abdomen, near the midline. He said the pain usually started 1 to 4 hours after a meal and sometimes awakened him at night. He also said that eating and antacids relieved the pain. He expressed concern that he had cancer.

Nursing diagnosis	Nursing objectives	Nursing actions

c MINI-SITUATION: Arthur Stewart, an unmarried black construction worker, was surprised to learn at a routine on-the-job physical examination that he had essential hypertension. He had a BP reading of 160/100. On interview, Mr. Stewart told the nurse that his father had died from a cerebral vascular accident at the age of 48. He also revealed he was a heavy cigarette smoker and daily ate "junk" food high in fat and calories.

Nursing diagnosis	Nursing objectives	Nursing actions

d MINI-SITUATION: Sarah Lutomski was admitted to the hospital in an acute asthma attack. She was having difficulty breathing and exhibited the characteristic asthmatic wheeze on expiration. She was perspiring profusely and appeared very tense and anxious.

Nursing diagnosis	Nursing objectives	Nursing actions

e MINI-SITUATION: Muriel Martin has a long history of rheumatoid arthritis. She experienced periods when she was relatively symptom free. At other times she experienced swollen and painful joints that limited her mobility. Applications of moist heat and the administration of salicylates provided some relief from pain. She was admitted to the medical service.

Nursing diagnosis	Nursing objectives	Nursing actions

DIRECTIONS: Select the *best* response. (Answers appear in the Appendix.)

1 The process whereby an individual's feelings, emotional needs, and/or conflicts are manifested through physical symptoms that have an organic basis is known as:

  a Hypochondriasis.   c Malingering.

  b Conversion.   d Somatization.

2 The obsolete designation psychosomatic illness has been replaced by the phrase psychophysiological disorders to reflect the current belief that these disorders are all:

  a Products of the client's imagination.

  b Based on psychological rather than physiological needs.

  c Caused by physical imbalance from emotional problems.

  d Reflections of the interrelationship between the mind and body.

3 Psychophysiological disorders are characterized by *all but which one* of the following?

  a Organic change in one body system.

  b Innervation by the central nervous system.

  c Underlying unconscious emotional conflicts.

  d Presence of anxiety over symptoms.

4 Which one of the following nursing objectives takes *priority* for a client admitted to the hospital with a bleeding peptic ulcer?

  a Restoring physiological homeokinesis.

  b Meeting client's dependency needs.

  c Encouraging the expression of feelings.

  d Decreasing the client's anxiety.

5 The personality of an individual prone to peptic ulcers is described as strong, self-sufficient, hardworking, and unemotional. Some theorists believe that these characteristics reflect a reaction formation to an unconscious conflict with:

  a Trust.   c Dependency.

  b Guilt.   d Love.

6 Persons with essential hypertension are often unaware that they have a physical problem or that they have huge amounts of repressed rage. The defense mechanism being utilized is frequently:

  a Denial.   c Conversion.

  b Suppression.   d Apathy.

7 The physiological factors contributing to the onset of bronchial asthma include:

  a Bacterial infection.   c Idiopathic bronchospasm.

  b Allergic reaction.   d All of the above.

8 The asthmatic wheeze is often described as a "cry for the mother." This interpretation reflects belief in the theory of:

  a Repressed conflicts.   c Symbolism.

  b Personality type.   d Organ weakness.

9 Which one of the following psychophysiological disorders involves the integumentary system?

    a Skin rashes.   c Bronchial asthma.

    b Rheumatoid arthritis.   d Ulcerative colitis.

10 The phrase "He's too thick-skinned" uses "body language" to express which one of the following emotions?

    a Insensitivity.   c Hostility.

    b Stubbornness.   d Suspiciousness.

11 Persons with rheumatoid arthritis are thought to have a superego that is essentially:

    a Permissive.   b Reasonable.   c Weak.   d Punitive.

12 Which one of the following theories *best* explains the "fight-or-flight" response in psychophysiological disorders?

    a Repressed-conflict theory.   c Symbolism theory.

    b Personality-type theory.   d Organ-weakness theory.

13 Which one of the following statements is *least* likely to be true of persons with a psychophysiological disorder?

    a They have unconscious emotional conflicts.

    b Their physical illness manifests organic changes.

    c They lose contact with reality when under stress.

    d Their physical illness serves to lower anxiety.

14 The primary gain associated with developing physical symptoms in response to stress is to:

    a Accept dependency.   c Experience attention.

    b Suppress anger.   d Decrease anxiety.

15 Minimizing secondary gains after the acute stage of illness can *best* be accomplished by which one of the following nursing actions?

    a Encouraging the client to take on responsibility for some aspects of his or her care.

    b Assuming a consistently sympathetic manner when with the client.

    c Anticipating the client's needs for the duration of his or her hospitalization.

    d Emphasizing the positive aspects of the illness, such as giving the client a needed rest.

16 Behaviors observed in psychophysiological disorders can be grouped around one of eight human processes. Which one of the following human processes is *least* likely to be affected in psychophysiological disorders?

    a Emotional processes.   c Interpersonal processes.

    b Cognition processes.   d Perception processes.

17 In conversation with the nurse, a client acutely ill with a psychophysiological disorder would be *most* likely to:

    a Focus on his or her inability to participate in self-care.

    b Discuss his or her failure in maintaining the home environment.

    c Explore his or her underlying emotional conflicts.

    d Express anxious feelings about his or her physical symptoms.

18 In planning care for clients with psychophysiological disorders, a short-term nursing objective would be to assist the client in regaining physiological homeokinesis. The *most* appropriate long-term nursing objective would be to help the client:

a Develop alternative coping measures.

b Resume home maintenance activities.

c Learn new diversional recreational patterns.

d Assume responsibility for self-care activities.

19 In communicating with clients with a psychophysiological disorder the nurse can be *most* therapeutic by:

a Giving them detailed information about their illness and care.

b Exploring the relationship between their physical symptoms and emotions.

c Encouraging them to talk about their feelings.

d Interpreting the symbolism behind their physical symptoms.

20 Which one of the following nursing actions would be *most* specific to the nursing diagnoses that state: Altered Self-Concept R/T unconscious conflicts between dependency and independency needs (ANA: 6.3.2) or Self-Esteem Disturbance R/T unconscious conflicts between dependency and independency needs (NANDA: 7.1.2)?

a Calling the client by his or her surname.

b Carrying out prescribed treatments.

c Responding with consistency at all times.

d Listening to the client's concerns.

19

Individuals with substance abuse and dependence

INTRODUCTION

"Very few human behaviors have consequences as far reaching as do those of the substance-dependent individual. In addition to affecting his own physical, emotional, and social well-being, the behavior of the substance-dependent individual affects the well-being of his family and that of the society at large." *
The problem of substance dependence is probably one of our greatest health problems, and the nurse encounters individuals with this problem in a wide variety of settings. With the exception of detoxification and rehabilitation centers and, most recently, medical services caring for individuals with drug-related acquired immune deficiency syndrome (AIDS) where nurses are directly involved on a consistent basis with the care of substance-dependent adults, many nurses may unwittingly be caring for individuals whose presenting problems are something else. In industry, for example, absenteeism and injuries may be related to drug or alcohol abuse. Similarly, individuals may be brought into general hospitals for physical problems related to drug or alcohol withdrawal, for accidental or intentional overdose, and for injuries sustained in automobile accidents as well as in domestic or other violent encounters while under the influence of an addicting agent. In schools increasing numbers of children and adolescents are being seen for poor performance and decreased productivity associated with substance dependence.

Adults with a substance dependence problem often evoke negative feelings in others based on personal experiences, stereotypes, and misconceptions. Several years ago a therapist who was supportive and therapeutic with most clients was heard exploding in frustration and anger at the manipulations of an alcoholic client. She subsequently revealed that her father had been an alcoholic and that she had never resolved her negative feelings toward substance-dependent individuals. Her feelings made it virtually impossible for her to respond therapeu-

---

*From Taylor CM: Mereness' essentials of psychiatric nursing, ed 13, St Louis, 1990, The CV Mosby Co, chap 19.

tically to them. At the time a student nurse who had identified himself as a recovering alcoholic and a member of Alcoholics Anonymous requested to work with the client and the staff. In the course of the nurse-client relationship the client experienced acceptance and understanding from the student. In a relatively brief time the client was also accepted and supported by most members of the staff, who developed a greater understanding of the problems and needs of alcoholic clients in general and this client in particular. Eventually the client was transferred to a facility supported by Alcoholics Anonymous that was more specifically designed to meet his special needs. The first step in this positive outcome was to identify negative feelings about alcohol use and about individuals who abuse alcohol. The second step was to then evaluate the effect negative feelings have on therapeutic intervention. If the therapist had not been willing to acknowledge her feelings of anger and helplessness and had not been willing to accept the help of another health care worker, the outcome in this situation might have been very different and probably not very therapeutic.

The exercises in this chapter are designed to help you increase your awareness of your feelings and attitudes toward individuals who abuse and are dependent on alcohol and/or drugs, to promote an increased understanding of these dysfunctional responses, and to apply selected phases of the nursing process to the care of substance-dependent individuals.

OBJECTIVES

1. To reflect on one's subjective responses to substance-dependent individuals as a step toward greater self-awareness.
2. To apply selected phases of the nursing process to clinical situations.
3. To evaluate selected treatment measures used in the care of substance-dependent individuals.

EXERCISES

1 What are your beliefs and attitudes toward the drinking of alcoholic beverages and the taking of drugs and toward individuals who engage in such activities?

   a Read each of the following ten attitudinal statements and indicate whether you agree or disagree with it, placing a check in the box in the appropriate column.

Attitudes	Agree	Disagree
1. Parents who drink and use drugs should hide the fact from their children.	☐	☐
2. Drinking two or three cocktails before dinner is an appropriate way to relax.	☐	☐
3. People who rely on drugs are weak-willed individuals.	☐	☐
4. Everyone should have a medicine cabinet well stocked with pills to meet any emergency.	☐	☐
5. Alcohol makes you sexy.	☐	☐
6. All drug addicts are criminals and should be punished.	☐	☐
7. It is appropriate to take sleeping pills whenever you cannot sleep.	☐	☐
8. Alcohol is a stimulant and helps pep you up.	☐	☐
9. All alcoholics are ineffectual human beings who should be pitied.	☐	☐
10. People who use alcohol or drugs in response to stress are morally inferior to other people.	☐	☐

b All of the previous statements reflect beliefs and attitudes toward persons who use alcohol and drugs to varying degrees. With how many did you agree? What other beliefs or attitudes do you have that are not included on this list?

c Share your responses with classmates and colleagues in a supervised classroom setting. The following questions are suggested to help focus the discussion.

1. What are the attitudes in your family toward the use of alcohol and drugs?
2. What cultural or religious factors may influence your attitudes toward substance use?
3. What experiences have you had with persons who have used alcohol or drugs to excess?
4. If your attitudes are essentially negative and nonaccepting, how would you feel about caring for a person with a substance-dependency problem?
5. How would you be able to control your feelings so as not to respond judgmentally while giving nursing care to these individuals?

2 The following list of ten nursing diagnoses is applicable to substance-dependent individuals. Using your knowledge of physiology, symptomatology, themes, dynamics, etc., make a brief statement about how or why each diagnosis applies. The first one has been filled in to help you get started.

a Altered Level of Consciousness R/T excessive use of alcohol (ANA: 7.6.2.1) or Confusion/Disorientation R/T excessive use of alcohol (ANA: 2.6.2.4) or Altered Thought Processes R/T excessive use of alcohol (NANDA: 8.3): At a level of 0.10% alcohol in the blood, motor and speech activity are impaired. With increasing intake of alcohol, additional deterioration of functioning is seen, including confusion and disorientation.

b Altered Sensory Perception R/T abrupt withdrawal of alcohol (ANA: 6.4.2) or Sensory/Perceptual Alterations R/T abrupt withdrawal of alcohol (NANDA: 7.2):

c Altered Social Interaction R/T unacceptable social behavior (ANA: 5.7.2) or Impaired Social Interaction R/T unacceptable social behavior (NANDA: 3.1.1):

d Altered Conduct/Impulse Processes R/T ineffective ego functions (impulse control) from excessive alcohol consumption (ANA: 5.3.2) or Potential for Violence (directed at others) R/T ineffective ego functions (impulse control) from excessive alcohol consumption (NANDA: 9.2.2):

e Altered Feeling State (Anxiety) R/T inaccessibility of alcohol and/or drugs on which individual is dependent (ANA: 4.1.2.2) or Anxiety R/T inaccessibility of alcohol and/or drugs on which individual is dependent (NANDA: 9.3.1):

f Altered Nutrition Processes R/T inadequate food and fluid intake (ANA: 7.7.2) or Altered Nutrition (less than body requirements) R/T inadequate food and fluid intake (NANDA: 1.1.2.2):

g Altered Judgment R/T excess intake of alcohol and/or mind-altering drugs (ANA: 2.2.2) or Decisional Conflict R/T excess intake of alcohol and/or mind-altering drugs (NANDA: 5.3.1.1):

h Altered Sensory Perception R/T use of hallucinogens (ANA: 6.4.2) or Sensory/Perceptual Alterations R/T use of hallucinogens (NANDA: 7.2):

i Suicide Attempt(s) R/T withdrawal of cocaine and/or crack (ANA: 5.3.2.9) or Potential for Violence (self-directed) R/T withdrawal of cocaine and/or crack (NANDA: 9.2.2):

j Altered Self Care R/T impairment from substance abuse (ANA: 1.3.4) or Bathing/Hygiene Self Care Deficit R/T impairment from substance abuse (NANDA: 6.5.2):

3 Read the following situations and, using the available data, develop nursing care plans reflecting the care Mr. White received at two different periods of his hospitalization. The nursing diagnoses and nursing objectives have been entered to help you get started.

a SITUATION: When Mr. White, jobless and a widower with four children, was discovered in a semiconscious state by his friends in Alcoholics Anonymous, he was taken to a general hospital and admitted to a unit maintained by Alcoholics Anonymous. Physical examination at the time of Mr. White's admission revealed many old and new bruises apparently sustained from falls while under the influence of alcohol. He was malnourished and dehydrated. He was disoriented in terms of time, place, and person. Mr. White was placed on bed rest in a single room. The atmosphere was quiet, the lighting subdued. He was assigned to a team of nurses who would provide him with consistency and continuity of nursing care twenty-four hours a day for the duration of his hospital stay. IV fluids were started. Anticonvulsant medications and B vitamins, specifically thiamine and niacin, were administered. Vital signs were taken, and he was found to have an elevation in temperature. Cooling measures were instituted. While carrying out their care, the nurses called Mr. White by name, told him who they were, and always oriented him to what they were doing.

Nursing Diagnosis #1: Altered Level of Consciousness R/T excessive and prolonged use of alcohol (ANA: 7.6.2.1) or Altered Health Maintenance R/T excessive and prolonged use of alcohol (NANDA: 6.4.2).

Nursing objective	Nursing actions	Anticipated outcomes
To help client regain physical homeostasis.		

184

b SITUATION: When Mr. White regained consciousness he was given oral fluids and placed on a diet high in protein and low in fat. The anticonvulsant medications and vitamins were continued. In addition he received an anxiolytic medication to help him through the period of alcohol withdrawal. He was ambulated gradually, but while he was in bed the side rails were used. He continued to be called by name and oriented to where he was and what had happened to him. The team of nurses assigned to him continued to provide consistency and continuity of care, seeking him out, sitting with him, and encouraging him to speak about himself and his concerns. Mr. White expressed a wide range of emotions: concern for his children, embarrassment at finding himself on an alcoholic unit, despair over his inability to manage himself and his life better, fear for the future. The nurses told him about the provisions that had been made for his children while he was hospitalized and arranged for them to visit him. Mr. White's friends from Alcoholics Anonymous visited daily for the two weeks that he was in the hospital. They, too, listened to his feelings and problems and identified ways that the organization and its members could assist him, including helping him find a job and reestablishing himself with his children.

Nursing Diagnosis #2: Altered Health Maintenance R/T excessive and prolonged use of alcohol (ANA: 1.3.4.4; NANDA: 6.4.2).

Nursing objective	Nursing actions	Anticipated outcomes
To help client regain physical homeostasis.		

Nursing Diagnosis #3: Altered Self Concept R/T feelings of despair, guilt, worthlessness (ANA: 6.3.2) or Self Esteem Disturbance R/T feelings of despair, guilt, worthlessness (NANDA: 7.1.2).

Nursing objective	Nursing actions	Anticipated outcomes
To help increase client's self-esteem.		

4 Symptomatology and nursing care may be grouped according to the ANA Classification of Human Responses of Concern for Psychiatric Mental Health Nursing Practice, Draft IV-R (September 20, 1988). In each of the following eight human processes, identify characteristic symptoms exhibited by a person dependent on narcotics and list examples of relevant nursing actions. The first one has been filled in to help you get started.

Human processes	Symptoms of narcotic dependency	Nursing actions
1. Activity processes.	Psychomotor retardation, activities focused on obtaining drugs, neglect of grooming.	1. Use patience and understanding when giving care. 2. Assist with grooming.
2. Cognition processes.		
3. Ecological processes.		
4. Emotional processes.		
5. Interpersonal processes.		
6. Perception processes.		
7. Physiological processes.		
8. Valuation processes.		

5 Substance-dependent individuals will generally exhibit symptoms of withdrawal when the addictive agent is no longer available. In the space below list twelve symptoms of withdrawal in narcotic-dependent individuals and six symptoms of withdrawal in alcohol-dependent individuals. One symptom has been filled in to help you get started.

Symptoms of narcotic withdrawal	Symptoms of alcohol withdrawal
1. Tearing	1.
2.	2.
3.	3.
4.	4.
5.	5.
6.	6.
7.	
8.	
9.	
10.	
11.	
12.	

6 Evaluate the following treatment programs used in the care of substance-dependent individuals.

a List three factors that have contributed to the success of Alcoholics Anonymous in the treatment of alcohol-dependent individuals.

1. _____

2. _____

3. _____

b List three advantages and three disadvantages of the methadone treatment program in the care of persons addicted to heroin.

Advantages:

1. _____

2. _____

3. _____

Disadvantages:

1. _____

2. _____

3. _____

DIRECTIONS: Select the *best* response. (Answers appear in the Appendix.)

1 The Volstead Act (1920) provided for which one of the following?
   a Making the sale of alcoholic beverages illegal.
   b Licensing physicians to dispense narcotics.
   c Regulating drug traffic in and out of the country.
   d Taxing cigarette and beer sales.

2 The term *tolerance* used in relation to substance dependence refers to which one of the following?
   a Individual's compulsive use of alcohol or drugs to achieve a sense of well-being.
   b Government's failure to act responsibly in controlling availability of alcohol and drugs.
   c Family's acceptance or indifference to a member's drug or alcohol-dependency problem.
   d Individual's need for increased amounts of alcohol or drugs to achieve the desired effect.

3 Which one of the following drugs is a synthetic substitute for opium?
   a Morphine.   c Codeine.
   b Heroin.   d Methadone.

4 Withdrawal symptoms for the heroin user include *all but which* one of the following?
   a Great irritability.   c Abdominal cramps.
   b Pinpoint pupils.   d Joint pain.

5 Methadone as a treatment for drug dependency is controversial mainly because it:
   a Is just as expensive as heroin.
   b Must be administered parenterally.
   c Maintains the individual's dependence on another drug.
   d Interferes with the individual's motivation to change.

6 A nursing action carried out prior to administering methadone to a person addicted to heroin is:
   a Checking the dietary intake.
   b Collecting a urine specimen.
   c Drawing blood for chemistries.
   d Taking all vital signs.

7 Some people describe alcohol as a "superego solvent," meaning that it removes the barriers to behavior normally provided by the superego. This phenomenon is *best* reflected in the statement that says that alcohol:
   a Encourages the expression of id impulses.
   b Releases an individual's learned inhibitions.
   c Interferes with judgment and impulse control.
   d Clouds an individual's memory for recent events.

8 Treatment for delirium tremens includes use of *all but which* one of the following?

    a Stimulants.   **c** Sedatives.

    b Anticonvulsants.   **d** Vitamins.

9 In which one of the following drug dependencies is it *absolutely essential* that the substance be withdrawn gradually?

    a Cocaine.   **c** LSD.

    b Heroin.   **d** Phenobarbital.

10 Which one of the following agents is *not* a central nervous system depressant?

    a Alcohol.   **c** Cocaine.

    b Barbiturates.   **d** Opiates.

11 Which of the following factors is said to be responsible for the fast and intense dependency that occurs among crack users?

    a Low cost.   **c** Intense euphoria.

    b Short duration of effect.   **d** All of the above.

12 The "street term" for amphetamines is:

    a Pot.   **c** Crack.

    b Speed.   **d** Acid.

13 The *most* commonly abused hallucinogen is:

    a Lysergic acid diethylamide.   **c** Phencyclidine.

    b Methamphetamine.   **d** Marijuana.

14 Characteristically, substance-dependent families are said to function by *all but which* one of the following guidelines?

    a Unrealistic rules of conduct.

    b Rigid rules discouraging change.

    c Rules rewarding positive behavior.

    d Rules prohibiting open communication.

15 Which one of the following defenses interferes the *most* with a person recognizing and accepting substance abuse as a problem?

    a Denial.   **c** Suppression.

    b Preoccupation.   **d** Regression.

16 Alcoholics Anonymous has been most effective treating individuals who abuse alcohol *primarily* because it:

    a Is readily available at a reasonable cost.

    b Meets the alcoholic's dependency needs.

    c Has a large, supportive membership.

    d Involves families in the care of their member.

17 Observation of psychomotor hyperactivity among substance-dependent individuals would suggest that they were abusing which of the following drugs?

    a Barbiturates.   **c** Amphetamines.

    b Opiates.   **d** All of the above.

18 Behavior observed in substance-dependent individuals can be grouped around one of eight human processes. Which one of the following behaviors reflects alteration of valuation processes?

a Ataxia.

b Euphoria.

c Powerlessness.

d Impulsiveness.

19 Which one of the following nursing actions would be *most* specific to the nursing diagnosis that states: Altered Conduct/Impulse Processes R/T weak ego (ANA: 5.3.2)?

a Listening to clients' verbal expressions of anger.

b Identifying to clients the consequences of their behavior.

c Focusing and acknowledging clients' strengths.

d Allowing clients to focus at length on past problems.

20 Which one of the following nursing objectives takes priority when caring for an individual with substance abuse problems?

a To regain physiological homeokinesis.

b To increase feelings of self-esteem.

c To develop functional methods of coping with stress.

d To relate to people who do not engage in substance abuse.

20 Individuals with personality disorders

Individuals with personality disorders are often maligned by the general public. In addition, professional and nonprofessional caretakers alike sometimes fail to recognize that adults whose behaviors are socially disruptive are human beings with unique problems. These responses, by the lay public and professionals alike, are often the result of negative personal experiences such as having been manipulated or otherwise used by a person with a personality disorder and/or the result of hearsay from others who may have been similarly victimized. Basically, however, these negative responses occur because of a lack of understanding.

"The causative factors of personality disorders are essentially unknown."* Although the behaviors exhibited by these individuals are generally believed to characterize earlier eras of life, why these fixations occur remains a mystery. Although generally accepted and considered normal in children (reflecting stages of development and an immature personality structure), observing these behaviors in adults evokes feelings of confusion, anger, fear, and avoidance; none of these feelings are conducive to the feelings of acceptance, respect, and consideration necessary for therapeutic intervention.

Individuals with personality disorders generally lack the insight and motivation to seek treatment for this disorder alone. With the exception of individuals with borderline personality and individuals with antisocial personality, most individuals with personality disorders are rarely hospitalized in psychiatric settings. They are, however, susceptible to physical problems and may well be encountered by nurses in other health-care settings. It is appropriate for all nurses to be able to assess the behaviors exhibited by these individuals, to be aware of any negative feelings they may experience in the course of carrying out nursing care, and to be alert to their clients' problems and needs so that they can carry out therapeutic holistic nursing care.

---

*From Taylor CM: Mereness' essentials of psychiatric nursing, ed 13, St Louis, 1990, The CV Mosby Co, chap 20.

The exercises in this chapter are designed to help you reflect on your feelings and attitudes toward individuals whose behaviors are socially disruptive as the first step toward greater self-awareness and therapeutic effectiveness. In addition, the exercises should help you to increase your understanding of these individuals and to apply selected phases of the nursing process to the care of these clients.

OBJECTIVES

1. To reflect on one's attitudes towards individuals whose behaviors are socially disruptive.
2. To apply selected phases of the nursing process to the care of adults whose behavior is socially disruptive.
3. To analyze ego functioning in individuals with antisocial personality disorder.

EXERCISES

1 To create a therapeutic interpersonal environment in which to treat adults whose behaviors are socially disruptive, nurses and other health care workers need to be aware of any negative attitudes they have towards such individuals.

a Listed below are ten statements reflecting negative attitudes about such individuals. Read each statement, decide whether you agree or disagree with it, and then place a check in the box in the appropriate column.

Attitudes	Agree	Disagree
Individuals with personality disorders:		
1. Should be imprisoned to protect society.	☐	☐
2. Could control their sexual impulses if they wanted to.	☐	☐
3. Are hopeless and trying to treat them is a waste of time and money.	☐	☐
4. Should not be hospitalized with mentally ill persons who may be victimized by them.	☐	☐
5. Are all criminals and deserve to be punished.	☐	☐
6. Should be castrated if they act out sexually.	☐	☐
7. Are all manipulative and not to be trusted.	☐	☐
8. Would be better off dead if they are self-destructive.	☐	☐
9. Deserve to be ostracized by society.	☐	☐
10. Are all "con artists" who will always use others to meet their needs.	☐	☐

b All of those statements are subjective responses to socially dysfunctional behaviors that can interfere with effective nursing activities. With how many did you agree?

c Share your feelings and beliefs with classmates and colleagues in a supervised classroom setting. The following questions are suggested to help focus the discussion:

1. Can you identify the source of your feelings? (Example: a past experience, something you have read, seen, or heard.)
2. What effect would communicating any of these feelings or beliefs to a person whose behavior is socially disruptive have on your efforts to develop a nurse-client relationship?
3. What can you do to begin to overcome these feelings and beliefs now that you are more aware of them?

2 Listed below are the eight human processes under which symptomatology and nursing care may be organized according to the ANA Classification of Human Responses of Concern for Psychiatric Mental Health Nursing Practice, Draft IV-R (September 20, 1988). In the space provided, describe at least one behavior and one nursing action specific to each one of the processes that are characteristically exhibited by individuals with a borderline personality disorder. Material for the first one has been filled in to help you get started.

Human processes	Behaviors	Nursing actions
1. Activity processes	Impulsive, substance abuse, sexual promiscuity, impatience, irritability.	Prevent impulsive motor behavior, teach socially acceptable ways of expressing emotion.
2. Cognition processes		
3. Ecological processes	Not applicable.	
4. Emotional processes		
5. Interpersonal processes		
6. Perception processes		
7. Physiological processes		
8. Valuation processes		

3 Marvin Wynter, a 32-year-old man, was admitted to the psychiatric service with a diagnosis (DSM-III-R) of Antisocial Disorder (301.70). A nursing diagnosis of Altered Conduct/Impulse Processes R/T inadequate ego development and functioning (ANA: 5.3.2) was made based on assessment data and an analysis of his behaviors. Although his ego does function effectively to a limited degree, which is reflected by a good memory, high intelligence, and an awareness of reality, it is ineffective in several areas.

a Listed below are fifteen behaviors observable in Mr. Wynter and indicative of a dysfunctional ego. A behavior may reflect more than one such dysfunction. Read each behavior and place a check in the box or boxes in the appropriate ineffective ego function column(s). The first one has been filled in to help you get started.

Behaviors	Ineffective ego functions				
	Ineffective use of cognitive abilities	Dysfunctional relationships with others	Lack of insight, judgment	Failure to control impulses	Failure to develop mature identification with others
1. Uses his charm to "con" others.	☑	☑	☐	☐	☐
2. Drinks heavily, then drives his car.	☐	☐	☐	☐	☐
3. Writes checks he cannot cover.	☐	☐	☐	☐	☐
4. Associates with persons living on the "fringe of society."	☐	☐	☐	☐	☐
5. Loses his temper easily and acts out violently.	☐	☐	☐	☐	☐
6. Denies that he has any emotional problems.	☐	☐	☐	☐	☐
7. Fabricates (lies) to cover his misdeeds.	☐	☐	☐	☐	☐
8. Exhibits dysfunctional behaviors characteristic of his father.	☐	☐	☐	☐	☐
9. Blames others for his "misfortunes."	☐	☐	☐	☐	☐
10. Manipulates others for profit.	☐	☐	☐	☐	☐
11. Justifies stealing and cheating with rationalizations.	☐	☐	☐	☐	☐
12. Spends money irresponsibly.	☐	☐	☐	☐	☐
13. Acts out impulsively with no concern for consequences.	☐	☐	☐	☐	☐
14. Maintains few loyalties.	☐	☐	☐	☐	☐
15. Adopts the substance abuse pattern observed in his mother.	☐	☐	☐	☐	☐

b Develop a nursing care plan for Mr. Wynter, listing four to five nursing actions and several outcome criteria appropriate to the stated nursing objective. One nursing action has been filled in to help you get started.

Nursing objective	Nursing actions	Outcome criteria
To help client develop impulse control.	Use a contract and identify behavioral expectations.	

TEST ITEMS

DIRECTIONS: Select the *best* response. (Answers appear in the Appendix.)

1 The terms *sociopathic* and *psychopathic* are obsolete labels for persons now identified as:
  a Antisocial.
  b Borderline.
  c Histrionic.
  d Narcissistic.

2 Paranoid, schizoid, and schizotypal personality disorders are *best* characterized by behaviors considered:
  a Emotional or erratic.
  b Manipulative or controlling.
  c Anxious or fearful.
  d Odd or eccentric.

3 Persons with borderline personality disorder are characterized by which of the following?
  a Failure to develop an integrated sense of self.
  b Fear of being alone.
  c Extreme mood shifts over short periods of time.
  d All of the above.

4 Which one of the following *most* characterizes individuals with antisocial personality disorder?
  a Anticipatory anxiety.
  b Charismatic personality.
  c Criminal behavior.
  d Sexual acting-out.

5 A person who consciously fabricates stories to impress others and to get out of compromising situations is:

   a Rationalizing.   c Projecting.

   b Cheating.   d Lying.

6 The individual with a personality disorder differs from the professional criminal in that the professional criminal's responses are characterized by:

   a Compulsive acts of criminal activity and aggressiveness.

   b Impulsivity and low tolerance for frustration.

   c Careful, long-range planning of criminal activity.

   d Obsessive thoughts focused on outwitting others.

7 Individuals with borderline personality disorder have been unable to develop a unified, integrated self-concept. The defense mechanism in operation is:

   a Undoing.   c Dissociation.

   b Splitting.   d Isolation.

8 Which part of the personality dominates persons with antisocial behaviors?

   a Id.   c Conscience.

   b Ego.   d Ego ideal.

9 The interpersonal relationships of individuals diagnosed with borderline personality disorder are *best* characterized as:

   a Intense.   c Superficial.

   b Brief.   d All of the above.

10 Which one of the following nursing care objectives is *most* specific to the care of individuals with borderline personality disorder?

   a Help client control impulsive behavior.

   b Help reduce the client's anxiety.

   c Help client develop emotional insight.

   d Help client rechannel testing behaviors.

11 The *most* effective nursing measure in response to acting-out behaviors is:

   a Setting limits on impulsive behavior.

   b Anticipating volatile situations.

   c Pointing out inappropriate behavior.

   d Accepting angry outbursts.

12 The self-mutilation frequently observed in clients with borderline personality commonly reflects:

   a Testing.   c Mimicking.

   b Splitting.   d All of the above.

13 The emotional processes of individuals with antisocial personality disorder are *best* characterized as:

   a Anxious.   c Shallow.

   b Remorseful.   d Bizarre.

14 Which one of the following nursing diagnoses is *least* applicable to the antisocial individual—Social Isolation (NANDA: 3.1.2) R/T?
   a Unaccepted social behavior.
   b Inability to engage in satisfying personal relationships.
   c Unaccepted social values.
   d Deficiency in intelligence.
15 In response to a client's manipulative behaviors the nurse should provide:
   a Reasonable punishment.   c Consistent limits.
   b Permissive atmosphere.   d Friendly manner.

21

Populations at risk
The elderly

INTRODUCTION

INTRODUCTION

"Most elderly persons are able to lead active and productive lives and continue to develop and learn during this developmental period. A person who has successfully completed earlier developmental tasks has a higher possibility of successfully completing the task of aging, and a helpful and supportive environment certainly contributes to its successful resolution." *

However, although people are living longer and healthier lives, problems do arise. A variety of physiological, social, psychological, and environmental stressors, in combination or alone, impinge on the elderly and create difficulties. Diminishing interpersonal and economic resources, decreasing physiological functions, increasing urbanization, accelerating rates of social change, and discriminating practices have increased their vulnerability and have indeed made them a "population at risk."

As the elderly population increases, so does our number of elderly health care recipients. The exercises in this chapter are designed to help you increase your understanding of the needs of the aged and to apply selected phases of the nursing process to the care of elderly clients.

OBJECTIVES

1. To differentiate among characteristic responses observed in the elderly.
2. To apply selected phases of the nursing process to the care of elderly clients.

---

*From Taylor CM: Mereness' essentials of psychiatric nursing, ed 13, St Louis, 1990, The CV Mosby Co, chap 21.

1 The life review, with a tendency to reminiscence, appears to be a nearly universal adaptive response in old age, facilitating the satisfactory closure to life. In addition to the life review, there are five other responses or themes associated with, but not unique to, aging: loneliness, loss and grief, suspicion, depression (despair), and dementia (confusion). In this exercise read each one of the following fifteen statements made by elderly, retired residents of a nursing home. Categorize each one in terms of the characteristic responses to aging by placing a check in the box in the appropriate column. The first one has been filled in to help you get started.

| | Responses to aging | | | | | |
Statements	Life review	Loneliness	Depression	Suspicion	Dementia	Loss—grief
1. "When I was a boy, we used to go fishing every Sunday afternoon after church."	☑	☐	☐	☐	☐	☐
2. "I must get up. Let me up. I have to get dressed or else I will be late for work."	☐	☐	☐	☐	☐	☐
3. "I wish I could hear what they are saying. I'm certain they are talking about me."	☐	☐	☐	☐	☐	☐
4. "My wife died 13 years ago, but I still get sad when I talk about her."	☐	☐	☐	☐	☐	☐
5. "I remember our first car. My brothers and I took turns cranking it up to get it started."	☐	☐	☐	☐	☐	☐
6. "There is nothing left to live for. I can't go on like this anymore. Life has no meaning."	☐	☐	☐	☐	☐	☐
7. "I feel so alone. There is no one I can talk to anymore."	☐	☐	☐	☐	☐	☐
8. "Help me shave. I want to look my best when my mother visits me tonight."	☐	☐	☐	☐	☐	☐
9. "Why are people laughing at me behind my back?"	☐	☐	☐	☐	☐	☐
10. "My children don't visit anymore. I wish they would bring my grandchildren to see me."	☐	☐	☐	☐	☐	☐
11. "Life is an effort. I might as well be dead."	☐	☐	☐	☐	☐	☐
12. "When I was a girl, my beaus would flock to my porch on a summer's night and serenade me."	☐	☐	☐	☐	☐	☐
13. "What I miss most about being here is not having my old dog. I had to put him to sleep. It still makes me sad."	☐	☐	☐	☐	☐	☐
14. "Bring me my boots and my horse! Get me my bugle. I must sound the charge."	☐	☐	☐	☐	☐	☐
15. "I have no interest in eating. I wish they would stop feeding me and let me die."	☐	☐	☐	☐	☐	☐

2 "Survival with esteem—not mere physical survival—is the goal of the aged person."* Although stated in the text as the goal of the aged, this statement is also an appropriate objective for anyone actively involved in the care of elderly clients. It reflects a holistic approach to client care. Failure to acknowledge this goal can result in the dehumanization of the client. In the following poem survival with esteem is clearly the goal of the elderly woman who silently admonishes the nurse, "Open your eyes nurse, open and see, not a crabbit old woman, look closer, see me." The nurse, on the other hand, has apparently focused all her attention on meeting the woman's physical needs and has lost

---

*From Taylor CM: Mereness' essentials of psychiatric nursing, ed 13, St Louis, 1990, The CV Mosby Co, chap 21.

sight of her emotional needs. She has failed to communicate interest in and respect for her client. Read the following poem and complete the exercises as directed:

Look closer*

What do you see nurse, what do you see?
What are you thinking when you look at me?
A crabbit old woman, not very wise
Uncertain of habit, with far away eyes,
Who dribbles her food, and makes not reply,
When you say in a loud voice, "I do wish you'd try!"
Who seems not to notice the things that you do,
And forever is losing a stocking or shoe.
Who, unresisting or not, lets you do as you will
With bathing and feeding, the long day to fill.
Is that what you're thinking, is that what you see?
Then open your eyes, you're not looking at me.
I'll tell you who I am as I sit here so still,
As I move at your bidding, as I eat at your will.
I am a small child of 10, with a father and mother,
Brothers and sisters who love one another.
A young girl at 16 with wings at her feet
Dreaming that soon now a lover she'll meet.
A bride soon at 20, my heart gives a leap
Remembering the vows that I promised to keep.
At 25 now I have young of my own
Who need me to build a secure happy home.
A woman of 30, my young now grow fast,
Bound to each other with ties that should last.
At 40 my young now soon will be gone,
But my man stays beside me to see I don't mourn.
At 50 once more babies play around my knee,
Again we know children, my loved one and me.
Dark days are upon me, my husband is dead,
I look at the future, I shudder with dread,
For my young are all busy rearing young of their own.
And I think of the years and the love I have known.
I'm an old lady now and nature is cruel,
'Tis her jest to make old age look like a fool.
The body it crumbles, grace and vigor depart,
And now there is a stone where I once had a heart.
But inside this old carcass a young girl still dwells,
And now and again my battered heart swells.
I remember the joys, I remember the pain,
And I am loving and living life over again.
I think of the years all too few, gone so fast,
And accept the stark fact that nothing can last.
So open your eyes nurse, open and see,
Not a crabbit old woman, look closer, see me.

---

*From McCormack PM: Look closer (Crabbit old woman), J Gerontol Nurse 2:9, 1976.

a According to Erikson, the task of the elderly is ego integrity versus despair. Using the assessment phase of the nursing process, analyze the woman's response to aging in terms of her negotiation of the task of old age.

b Using the evaluation phase of the nursing process, identify three responses made by the nurse that were nontherapeutic and had a dehumanizing effect on the client.

1. _____

_____

2. _____

_____

3. _____

_____

c List below three behavioral responses seen in the elderly client that reflect dehumanization.

1. _____

_____

2. _____

_____

3. _____

_____

d Listed on p. 202 are selected verbal responses made by the elderly woman that reflect the characteristics and themes of aging. The themes are identified in parentheses. A nursing goal has been entered for each one. In the space provided revise the care that was given and list at least three nursing actions appropriate to each goal. One nursing action has been filled in to help you get started.

Behavioral responses/themes	Nursing goals	Nursing actions
1. "What do you see nurse, what do you see, what are you thinking when you look at me? A crabbit old woman, not very wise. . . " (Suspicion)	Facilitate communication and validation.	1. Initiate a nurse-client relationship. 2. 3. 4.
2. "Who seems not to notice the things that you do, and forever is losing a stocking or shoe." (Dementia)	Provide reality orientation and stimulation.	1. 2. 3.
3. "Dark days are upon me, my husband is dead, I look at the future, I shudder with dread." (Grief)	Encourage expression of feelings.	1. 2. 3.
4. "I look at the future, I shudder with dread, For my young are all busy rearing young of their own." (Loneliness)	Provide opportunities to relate.	1. 2. 3.
5. "I'm an old lady now and nature is cruel, 'tis her jest to make old age look like a fool." (Depression)	Increase self-esteem.	1. 2. 3.
6. "I remember the joys, I remember the pain, and I am loving and living life over again." (Life review)	Support the client in her reminiscences.	1. 2. 3.

3 Listed below are six nursing diagnoses that are applicable to elderly persons with behavioral disturbances. Using your knowledge of behaviors, signs and symptoms, themes, and dynamics, make a brief statement about how or why each diagnosis applies. The first one has been filled in to help you get started.

a Social Isolation (NANDA: 3.1.2) or Altered Social Interaction (ANA: 5.7.2) R/T inadequate personal resources: Loss of friends through illness, death, etc., plus decreased involvement with family, accounts for much of the social isolation experienced by the elderly.

b Potential for Violence: Self-Directed (NANDA: 9.2.2) or Suicidal Ideation (ANA: 5.3.2.10) R/T feelings of hopelessness and despair:

c Knowledge Deficit: Recent Events (NANDA: 8.1.1) or Short-Term Memory Loss (ANA: 2.5.2.5) R/T the life review:

d Self-Esteem Disturbance (NANDA: 7.1.2) or Altered Self-Concept (ANA: 6.3.2) R/T progressive deterioration of mental functioning:

e Bathing/Hygiene Self-Care Deficit (NANDA: 6.5.2) or Altered Self-Care (ANA: 1.3.4) R/T memory deficit:

f Sensory/Perceptual Alterations: Suspiciousness (NANDA: 7.2) or Altered Sensory Perception: Suspiciousness (ANA: 6.4.2.1) R/T difficulties negotiating the developmental task of trust:

4 Listed below are the eight human processes under which symptomatology and nursing care may be organized according to the ANA Classification of Human Responses of Concern for Psychiatric Mental Health Nursing Practice, Draft IV-R (September 20, 1988). In the space provided describe at least one behavior and one nursing action specific to each one of the processes that are characteristically exhibited by individuals who are victims of Alzheimer's disease. Material for the first one has been filled in to help you get started.

Human processes	Behaviors	Nursing actions
1. Activity processes	Activity intolerance, psychomotor agitation, gait impairment, decreasing involvement in self-care, sleeplessness, wandering.	Encourage client to carry out self-care as long as possible; warm baths, soft music, light exercise, small amount of wine at bedtime; close supervision to prevent wandering; antipsychotic medication as prescribed for agitation.
2. Cognition processes		
3. Ecological processes		
4. Emotional processes		
5. Interpersonal processes		
6. Perception processes		
7. Physiological processes		
8. Valuation processes		

DIRECTIONS: Select the *best* response. (Answers appear in the Appendix.)

1 Which of the following factors has contributed to the increased life expectancy and the growing number of elderly in the population?
   a Better preventive measures in health maintenance.
   b More effective treatment measures during illness.
   c Improved treatment of injuries.
   d All of the above.

2 Recent research indicates that mental problems of the elderly are primarily the result of:
   a Alzheimer's disease.   c Schizophrenia.
   b Anxiety disorders.   d Loneliness.

3 Which one of the following experiences has the *most* profound affect on the aged person?
   a Decreasing psychomotor abilities.
   b Increasing perceptual difficulties.
   c Diminishing income from retirement.
   d Failing memory for recent events.

4 The life review primarily involves which one of the following?
   a Grief.   c Depression.
   b Reminiscence.   d Loneliness.

5 Rather than grieve over interpersonal losses, many elderly people respond by:
   a Experiencing high anxiety.
   b Becoming very depressed.
   c Withdrawing from reality.
   d Developing physical symptoms.

6 In responding helpfully to the elderly client who painfully talks about guilty feelings associated with a significant loss that occurred years before, the nurse would do which of the following?
   a Validate to the client that it is painful to lose a loved one.
   b Introduce a neutral and less emotional topic to the client.
   c Reassure the client that there is no reason for feeling guilty.
   d All of the above.

7 Which one of the following responses to aging is *most* associated with Alzheimer's disease?
   a Suspiciousness.   c Reminiscence.
   b Dementia.   d Depression.

8 Which one of the following motor behaviors is a late symptom seen in clients with Alzheimer's disease?
   a Psychomotor retardation.   c Unsteady gait.
   b Altered self-care.   d Sleeplessness.

9 Individuals with Alzheimer's disease experience social isolation and withdrawal early in their illness because they are:

a Shunned by other people because of their bizarre behavior.

b Unable to recognize their friends and family members.

c Angry at being treated in a condescending manner.

d Embarrassed by their progressive deterioration.

10 Which one of the following is a physical problem that affects an individual with Alzheimer's disease during the *entire* course of the illness?

a Incontinence.   c Sleeplessness.

b Injury.   d Anorexia.

11 The valuation processes of individuals with Alzheimer's disease are characterized by which of the following?

a Helplessness.   c Powerlessness.

b Hopelessness.   d All of the above.

12 Which one of the following nursing care objectives is *most* specific to the care of victims of Alzheimer's disease?

a Help the client develop emotional insight.

b Help the client maintain mental acuity.

c Help the client control impulsive behavior.

d Help the client develop feelings of self-esteem.

13 Which one of the following nursing actions takes *priority* when giving care to a client with advanced Alzheimer's disease?

a Promoting group social interactions.

b Encouraging expressions of feelings.

c Providing safety measures.

d Facilitating the life review.

14 Antipsychotic medications are given to relieve extreme restlessness in persons with Alzheimer's disease. These medications are given in small amounts because of the:

a Weight loss commonly seen in the elderly.

b Delay in drug elimination from the body in the aged.

c Danger of suicide by overdosing in older people.

d Potentiation effect when taken with other drugs by the aged.

15 The Alzheimer's Disease and Related Disorders Association provides victims of Alzheimer's disease and their families with which of the following?

a Hot lines.   c Self-help groups.

b Respite care programs.   d All of the above.

22

Populations at risk
Children and adolescents

Like adults, children and adolescents respond with characteristic behaviors when they are unable to cope with the developmental tasks and the challenges posed by a complex and postindustrial society. Suffering from severe stress, they may be overwhelmed and seek to escape through self-destructive acts such as suicide attempts, substance abuse, and eating disorders. They may seek refuge in disorders commonly seen in adults, such as psychotic, somatic, and anxiety disorders. Rather than talk about their emotions of fear, anxiety, and despair, they may manifest temper tantrums, enuresis, thumb sucking, clinging, and other regressive behaviors. They may also act out in truancy, juvenile delinquency, sexual promiscuity, and aggressiveness. Today's runaways reflect troubled and highly vulnerable youth. These dysfunctional behaviors all serve the same dual purpose in young people as they do in adults, that is, to communicate distress and to reduce severe anxiety.

With the advances in medical science, infants born with multiple genetic defects, including brain dysfunction and cognitive impairment, are surviving well into the childhood, adolescent, and adult years. These persons constitute a growing population with multiple physical and emotional needs that must be recognized and met. In addition, their physical and cognitive problems make them particularly vulnerable to the development of emotional illness. In providing care for them, nurses must take the intellectual limitations of this population into consideration.

One can readily say that "there probably is no other group for which the title 'Populations at Risk' is more appropriate than the group represented by the children and adolescents of this country. About one-third of the nation's population is under 18 years of age, and it is estimated that over 11% of this group is suffering from a mental disorder. Furthermore, many authorities forecast that the incidence and prevalence of mental disorders and dysfunctional behavior among this population will increase over the next two decades. Despite this dire situation, there is a gross shortage of health care professionals who are educationally and experientially prepared to address these problems. The seriousness of this situation can be appreciated if one remembers that the children and youth of a society are that society's future." *

Although the identification and care of mentally disturbed and cognitively impaired children and adolescents is generally considered a specialty, it is important that all nurses have some awareness of the scope of the problem and some understanding of the nursing care of these young people. The exercises in this chapter are designed to help you reflect on your feelings about disturbed children and adolescents as a step toward greater self-awareness and to apply phases of the nursing process to this "population at risk."

OBJECTIVES

1. To reflect on one's responses to emotionally disturbed and cognitively impaired children and adolescents.
2. To define mental retardation.
3. To differentiate between the four different categories of mental retardation.
4. To apply selected phases of the nursing process to the care of young people whose behaviors are dysfunctional.

EXERCISES

1 Self-awareness is an integral part of all phases of the nursing process. Beginning with assessment, when initial contact with a client is made, and ending with evaluation, when you look at the outcomes of your care, you need to focus on your feelings about working with a young person. Although true for all nurses, self-awareness may have particular relevance for young nurses who may be close in age to their adolescent clients and for all nurses who may have children similar in age to the clients with whom they are working. The purpose of this exercise is to help you engage in self-assessment. The following list of twelve topics is suggested for discussion, sharing of feelings, elaboration of personal experiences, and role-playing in a supervised group setting with colleagues and peers. You may be able to add other topics for discussion as you begin to work with young clients who are mentally retarded and/or emotionally disturbed. The success of this exercise is dependent on your willingness to share your feelings in the group and on your peers' ability to respond with respect and sensitivity to the feelings being shared.

a The client is manipulating one staff member against another to try and get special privileges to watch TV. You discover that the client has succeeded in manipulating you to give him these privileges, and you feel angry toward him.

b The client has a diagnosis of bulimia nervosa with episodes of binge feeding and purging. You come from a background where food was often scarce, and you feel that this client's behavior is wasteful and sinful.

---

*From Taylor CM: Mereness' essentials of psychiatric nursing, ed 13, St Louis, 1990, The CV Mosby Co, chap 22.

c The client is a young, good-looking man whom you find attractive. He invites you on a date and you feel in conflict.

d The client is a young, seductive woman whom you find attractive. She has aroused your sexual feelings and you feel guilty.

e The client is an anorexic adolescent girl who is emaciated. Her physical appearance is repulsive to you, and you are finding it difficult to accept her and respond in a caring way.

f The client is a young teenage boy who uses heroin. You have recently been robbed by a drug addict and feel angry toward this client even though he was not involved in your losses.

g The client is a young child who reminds you of your own children and evokes a variety of feelings (love, anger, guilt, etc.) that are interfering with your objectivity.

h The client is a teenage girl who has made several unsuccessful suicide attempts. She comes from a family that is well-off financially and has had many of the opportunities denied to a close friend or family member you know who succeeded in taking his own life. You are finding it difficult to respond in an understanding and accepting way to this young person.

i The client is hospitalized on a medical unit for care of physical problems associated with severe mental retardation. Your community is considering opening a group home for cognitively handicapped persons next door to your house. You are ambivalent about this and are having difficulty caring for this mentally retarded client.

j The client is a pregnant, unwed runaway who is debating whether or not to have an abortion. She has decided that she will not keep the baby should she carry it to term. Your religious and ethical values are making it difficult for you to respond therapeutically to this client.

k The client is very depressed. You too have been feeling depressed and associating with this client intensifies your feelings. You find yourself identifying with this client, and this is making it increasingly difficult for you to respond objectively.

l The client is an autistic child who exhibits temper tantrums, head-banging, and problems communicating verbally. You are the product of a strict home and feel the child is spoiled and willful. Your feelings are affecting your being able to give therapeutic care.

2 Define mental retardation.

3 Intelligence testing is one of the primary tools used to identify and categorize individuals who are mentally retarded. A score called the intelligence quotient (IQ) is calculated using the following formula:

$$IQ = \frac{MA \text{ (mental age)}}{CA \text{ (chronological age)}} \times 100$$

In the following four mini-situations each individual's intelligence quotient has been determined. Identify the degree of severity (mild, moderate, severe, or profound) and describe the characteristics of the levels of severity.

Mini-situations	Degree of severity	Characteristics
1. Aaron had been described as "slow" by his mother. However, he was not given an IQ test until he was 13 years old. At that time his IQ was determined to be 65.		
2. Suzy, a 5-year-old child, was taken by her mother to the developmental clinic because she felt the child was unresponsive. She was tested and found to have an IQ of 48.		
3. Joan suffered brain damage in a car accident. Her IQ following the accident was between 35 and 40.		
4. Bobby was diagnosed as being mentally retarded at birth. He had multiple genetic defects and anomalies. When he was 3 years old, he was tested, and his IQ was found to be below 20.		

4 Read the following eight mini-situations and write at least one appropriate nursing diagnosis for each one. Use the ANA and/or NANDA formats. One nursing diagnosis has been filled in to help you get started.

Mini-situations	Nursing diagnosis
1. Jeremy exhibited many behavioral problems in childhood— truancy, fire-setting, and shoplifting. At age 15 he raped his sister because "voices" told him to do it. He was hospitalized on a psychiatric service for observation. There was question, however, as to whether he was really psychotic or was using hallucinations to cover his inability to control his impulsive acts.	Altered Conduct/Impulse Processes R/T poor impulse control (ANA:5.3.2.) ....
2. Sarah's family traveled a good deal while Sarah was growing up. Consequently, she formed few friendships. When she was 16, her father died, and she and her mother settled down with her grandparents. Sarah attended high school and became involved with a peer group that was experimenting with drugs partly out of rebellion against authority and partly as a means to finding their identities. Sarah experienced a "bad trip" on LSD and was hospitalized because of severe anxiety, agitation, and violence directed toward herself and others.	
3. Alice has bulimia nervosa. She was admitted to the medical service and intravenous therapy was ordered to correct a severe electrolyte imbalance. On interview it was learned that Alice engaged in secret binge and purge episodes. She was aware that her preoccupation with food and dieting and the episodic binges followed by self-induced vomiting were not normal, and she concealed her activities from her family and friends. However, the repeated and unexplained disappearance of large quantities of food in the household made her family suspicious, and when Alice had to be hospitalized for dehydration and electrolyte imbalance, her behavior patterns and preoccupations were revealed.	
4. Deborah was diagnosed as being severely mentally retarded when she was a young child. She lived at home with her parents and sister until she was 8 years old. Then her parents sought professional help to deal with her multiple problems. Deborah was admitted to a developmental center for evaluation. At that time she was found to have minimal verbal skills and was unable to meet even her most basic hygiene needs.	

Continued.

Mini-situations	Nursing diagnosis
5. There had been several successful and near-successful suicides at Mike's school. In the aftermath of the anger and grief over these tragic events, parent, teacher, and student groups mobilized their efforts to learn about suicide and how to prevent it. Therefore, when Mike was denied admission to the college of his choice and subsequently offered his car to his best friend and a treasured record collection to his brother, his family, friends, and teachers were sensitive to his depression and suicidal ideation and arranged for him to receive professional help.	
6. Wayne had always been a neat child. When the other children engaged in artwork, sports, or other activities that might get him dirty, he hung back and would not participate. His mother was assured it was a phase that he would outgrow. Instead of outgrowing it, Wayne's preoccupation with cleanliness, order, dirt, and pollution increased. He was taken for professional help when his obsessions and ritualistic cleaning activities interfered with his school attendance.	
7. Cheryl refused to go to school and stayed in bed with the covers pulled up over her head. She was nonverbal. She used the bathroom but refused to eat her meals with the family. Food left on a tray in her room disappeared and her mother assumed she was eating. After a month, Cheryl was admitted for treatment to an adolescent unit in the state hospital.	
8. At age four, Geoffry was referred by the child care clinic to a facility specializing in the diagnosis and treatment of emotionally disturbed children. On interview his mother described her son as being very unresponsive to her as well as other people. She said he appeared to live in a private world. Although she said he could speak words, he did not use them in a meaningful way. Geoffry was diagnosed as suffering from autism.	

5 Clients diagnosed as having anorexia or bulimia nervosa clearly need care that is holistic in nature. Their physical and emotional problems are closely intertwined. In the following exercise, plan care for clients experiencing these eating disorders. A nursing diagnosis and nursing goals aimed at both their physical and emotional needs have been entered to help you get started. List nursing actions appropriate to each of the goals.

a Client with anorexia nervosa

Nursing diagnosis: Altered Nutrition: Less than body requirements R/T fear of fat and distorted body image (NANDA:1.1.2.2.) or Altered Eating Processes R/T fear of fat and distorted body image (ANA:1.4.2.2.).

Nursing goals	Nursing actions
1. Restoration of normal nutritional status.	
2. Promotion of feelings of self-esteem and self-worth.	

b Client with bulimia nervosa

Nursing diagnosis: Altered Health Maintenance R/T binge and purge episodes (NANDA: 6.4.2; ANA:1.3.4.4.)

Nursing goals	Nursing actions
1. Restoration of normal nutritional status.	
2. Promotion of feelings of self-esteem and self-worth.	

DIRECTIONS: Select the *best* response. (Answers appear in the Appendix.)

1 Historically, which one of the following events contributed *most* to an increased interest in childhood and adolescence as stages of development distinct from adulthood?

a Post World War II *baby boom*.

b Emergence of the industrial society.

c Community mental health movement.

d Child labor laws.

2 The diagnosis of mental retardation is *primarily* based on an assessment of which one of the following factors?

a Physical endowment. **c** Emotional expressions.

b Cognitive functioning. **d** Cultural background.

3 Which one of the following formulas is used to determine an individual's intelligence quotient (IQ)?

a CA/MA × 10.

b MA/CA × 100.

c CA/100 × MA.

d MA/10 × CA.

4 Individuals with an IQ of 35 to 55 (moderate degree of severity) should be able to achieve *all but which one* of the following levels of functioning?

a Communicate verbally.

b Meet basic hygiene needs.

c Function in unskilled jobs.

d Benefit from educational programs.

5 Factors contributing to the development of mental retardation include:

a Head injury at birth.

b Substance abuse by mother during pregnancy.

c Ingestion of toxins by the infant.

d All of the above.

6 Which one of the following behaviors is *most* specifically associated with autistic children?

a Clinging.

b Masturbating.

c Twirling.

d Lying.

7 Which one of the following nursing diagnoses using the ANA format would be *most* specific to an overactive child?

a Altered Attention R/T distractability (6.1.1).

b Altered Sexuality Patterns R/T lack of guilt (5.6.7).

c Altered Social Interaction R/T anxiety (5.7.2).

d Altered Student Role R/T impaired academic skills (5.5.2.4).

8 All disturbed children need an environment that provides opportunities for:

a Verbalization of concerns.

b Freedom of movement.

c Decision making.

d Ego development.

9 Emotionally disturbed children cared for in treatment centers are often exposed to several different health care workers. Which of the following therapeutic responses is the *most* difficult to provide?

a Empathy.

b Consistency.

c Reassurance.

d Love.

10 In responding to hyperactive children the nurse may need to provide reasonable limits. Which one of the following is the *most* effective way to restrain these children?

a Isolating them until the episode has subsided.

b Administering psychopharmacological agents as prescribed.

c Holding them firmly during the outburst.

d Verbalizing clear behavioral expectations.

11 Play therapy is employed in the treatment of disturbed children *primarily* to:

a Provide the children with insights into their unconscious conflicts.

b Allow the children to work through the problems they are experiencing.

c Help the children develop both their motor and social skills.

d Give the children opportunities to negotiate developmental tasks.

12 Which one of the following emotional disturbances is experienced by adolescents?

a Psychotic disorders.　　　　c Eating disorders.

b Substance abuse.　　　　　 d All of the above.

13 Which one of the following is associated with anorexia nervosa in its *early stages?*

a Distorted body image.　　　 c Amenorrhea.

b Loss of appetite.　　　　　　d Binge eating.

14 The individual with bulimia nervosa is characterized by *all but which one* of the following?

a Perfectionism.　　　　　　　c Severe dieting.

b Emaciation.　　　　　　　　 d Laxative abuse.

15 Which one of the following nursing diagnoses using the NANDA format *most* specifically reflects the problems of a person with bulimia nervosa?

a Altered Nutrition: Less than body requirements R/T fear of fat (1.1.2.2).

b Altered Health Maintenance R/T ineffective individual coping (6.4.2).

c Altered Health Maintenance R/T binge eating and purging behaviors (6.4.2).

d Altered Nutrition: More than body requirements R/T excessive food intake (1.1.2.1).

16 Which one of the following is the *most* appropriate short-term goal for a person with an eating disorder?

a To encourage client's expression of feelings.

b To restore client's normal nutritional status.

c To alter client's body image.

d To promote client's peer alliances.

17 Family dynamics contributing to adolescent suicide include which of the following?

a Family disorganization.　　　c Strict parental discipline.

b Lack of communication.　　　d All of the above.

18 Cues to adolescent suicide include:

a Giving away valued possessions.

b Talking about death and suicide.

c Changing sleep patterns.

d All of the above.

19 If the nurse suspects that an adolescent client is thinking about suicide, he/she should do which one of the following?

    a Introduce cheerful topics of conversation to distract him.

    b Avoid mentioning suicide to him to avoid precipitating a suicide attempt.

    c Encourage him to talk about his feelings and suicidal thoughts.

    d Tell him he should not commit suicide because it would hurt his family.

20 Which one of the following nursing actions would be *most* therapeutic for a person with poor body image and low self-esteem?

    a Telling her she is a worthwhile person.

    b Avoiding any form of criticism.

    c Encouraging a daily grooming routine.

    d Giving praise and compliments frequently.

23

Populations at risk
The physically ill

INTRODUCTION

Individuals confronted with a serious physical illness and hospitalization face a crisis. They and their families must adjust to a change in roles and life-style. Close, daily supportive relationships are usually disrupted by hospitalization. Self-esteem and body image may be threatened. Dehumanizing experiences are encountered. Privacy is invaded. Feelings of fear, anxiety, helplessness, hopelessness, and despair may be experienced.

One responds to a crisis precipitated by a physical illness in either an adaptive, growth-promoting way or in a dysfunctional, disorganizing way. Personality makeup, early life experiences, previous encounters with illness, and available coping measures all contribute to how the physically ill and their families respond when faced with serious illness, hospitalization, treatment measures, and the threat of possible death. In addition, the nature of the illness itself, whether acute or chronic, whether stigmatizing, disabling, disfiguring, or life-threatening, also plays a critical role in the behavioral outcomes manifested by this population at risk, the physically ill.

"It is a fact that current nursing care of persons who are physically ill is characterized by the execution of an increasing number of highly technical procedures, often to the neglect of attempts to meet the person's emotional needs."* Studies have indicated that growing dissatisfaction with nursing care is not related to physical care but rather to professional nurses' failure to establish meaningful, caring relationships with their clients. Nurses have been criticized for their impersonal approach and their lack of warmth and empathy. The following excerpt from the poem entitled *Efficient Care?*† illustrates this point all too well.

---

*From Taylor CM: Mereness' essentials of psychiatric nursing, ed 13, St Louis, 1990, The CV Mosby Co, chap 23.
†From Mezzanotte EJ: Efficient care? Nursing '74 4:37, 1974.

I am the proud recipient
Of fine intensive care.
Efficient, modern, monitored—
Describe my daily fare.

I cough. . . .I breathe. . . .I move. . . .I turn.
I'm like a small machine.
I've tubes and leads. I'm wired!! I'm tired!!
But God, I cannot sleep.

Will I live or will I die?
My prognosis is unknown.
Inside I'm tense. I ache. I quake.
I'm afraid to be alone.

I hear the sounds of busy feet
And feel the busy hands.
Voices that talk and seem concerned,
But do they understand?

Theoretically there is no dispute over the fact that physical needs take priority over emotional ones. This is clearly reflected in Maslow's *Hierarchy of Human Needs*. Practically speaking, however, the implementation of physical and emotional care can be carried out simultaneously by the skilled and sensitive nurse.

The exercises in this chapter are designed to help you focus on nursing activities that are effective in meeting the emotional needs of this population at risk, the physically ill. Since a clinical experience with physically ill clients is generally not part of a psychiatric nursing experience, it will be necessary for you to apply these learnings to clinical rotations involving physically ill individuals.

OBJECTIVES

1. To reflect on one's responses to physically ill individuals.
2. To apply selected phases of the nursing process to the care of individuals who are physically ill.
3. To review communication skills used to interact therapeutically with the dying client.
4. To describe the characteristics and behavioral responses associated with the five stages of dying.

EXERCISES

1 Clients' adaptations to the stress of physical illness, hospitalization, separation from family and friends, treatment measures, and the threat of death, often depend on helpful interactions with skilled and sensitive nurses. It is therefore important that nurses strive for self-awareness and be aware of their feelings about physically ill individuals, about their values of good and bad, of their judgments of right and wrong to provide optimum therapeutic care and meet the emotional needs of their physically ill clients. Listed on p. 220 are selected examples of physically ill clients that may elicit conflictual feelings in you and your peers. In a supervised classroom setting, share your feelings about these clients with your classmates and colleagues and discuss how these feelings may affect your care.

a Two clients were admitted to the intensive care unit with extensive second and third degree burns on the face and body. One was the arsonist who deliberately set the fire that injured the second client and also killed that client's wife. Do you feel differently about these two clients, and can you respond therapeutically to both of them?

b You are assigned to care for a 25-year-old client who was injured in an automobile accident. Upon examination he was found to be "brain dead." He is being kept alive on life-support systems against the family's wishes. How do you feel about sustaining life/terminating life when there is apparently no hope?

c Two clients share a semi-private room. Both have AIDS. One is a homosexual drug user and became infected through his life-style. The other client is a hemophiliac who became infected through a contaminated blood transfusion. How do you feel about caring for AIDS clients in general, these two clients in particular? Can you accept and treat both of them with understanding?

d The client is waiting for a suitable donor for a kidney transplant. The availability of dialysis to sustain the client while she waits is based on her ability to pay for the treatment. She is unable to finance the treatments and dies before a donor is found. How do you feel about the fairness of this system? Can you accept and treat objectively the client in the next room who is able to pay for her dialysis?

e Two clients are admitted for abortions. One is the victim of rape by her father. The other is a married career woman who decided that she was not yet ready to start a family. Do you feel differently about these two women and their right to terminate the life of their unborn child? How will your feelings affect your carrying out therapeutic nursing care with each of them?

f The client went through extensive head-and-neck surgery for cancer. Can you care for this client in an accepting way, or will his physical disfigurement make it difficult for you to look at him, let alone care for him, without feelings of revulsion?

2 Listed below and on p. 221 are seven nursing diagnoses using both the ANA and NANDA formats. Each diagnosis is specific to individuals who are physically ill. Using your knowledge of emotional reactions to physical illness, make a brief statement about how or why each diagnosis applies. The first one has been filled in to help you get started.

a Powerlessness R/T feelings of dehumanization from the use of life-sustaining mechanical devices (ANA:8.1.2.4; NANDA:7.3.2): Persons who depend on mechanical devices for life often feel that the devices are more important than they are, that they are part of the machine and have lost control over their bodies and their lives.

b Fear R/T organ transplants (ANA:4.1.2.4; NANDA:9.3.2):

c Altered Body Image R/T loss of a body part (ANA:6.3.2.1), Body Image Disturbance R/T loss of a body part (NANDA:7.1.1):

d Anger R/T dependency associated with long-term cardiac pathology and prospective cardiac surgery (ANA:4.1.2.1), Potential for Violence: Directed at Others R/T dependency associated with long-term cardiac pathology and prospective cardiac surgery (NANDA:9.2.2):

e Altered Self Esteem R/T the birth of an imperfect infant (ANA:6.3.2.3), Self Esteem Disturbance R/T the birth of an imperfect infant (NANDA:7.1.2):

f Altered Values R/T a successful planned abortion (ANA:8.3.2), Spiritual Distress R/T a successful planned abortion (NANDA:4.1.1):

g Social Isolation/Withdrawal R/T social ostracism and fear of transmission of/infection by the AIDS virus (ANA:5.7.2.5), Social Isolation R/T social ostracism and fear of transmission of/infection by the AIDS virus (NANDA:5.1.1).

3 Understanding, emotional support, realistic reassurance, acceptance, caring, empathy, and attentiveness are all general characteristics of therapeutic nursing responses. To be implemented with a client, each response must be expressed behaviorally. Specifically, what can the nurse do to show emotional support and acceptance? What can the nurse say to communicate caring and understanding?

List below six nursing approaches that behaviorally illustrate these general characteristics of therapeutic care. An example has been filled in to help you get started.

a Be alert to clients' verbal and nonverbal cues that indicate readiness to talk about themselves, their feelings, and their concerns.

b _____
_____
_____

c _____
_____
_____

d _____
_____
_____

e _____
_____
_____

f _____
_____
_____

g _____
_____
_____

4 Nurses caring for physically ill clients are faced with the possibility that the client may die. A sudden, unexpected death comes as a shock to everyone. The nurse may grieve along with the family. There is no opportunity to prepare for such a death or to work through feelings of loss in advance. A terminal illness in which death is anticipated, however, allows the client, the family, and the nurse to work through these feelings in advance of the death. This process is called anticipatory grief. Clients who are aware that they are dying often respond in a generally predictable pattern, going through five stages in the dying process: denial, anger, bargaining, depression (loss), and acceptance. Others involved with the dying person, including the family and the nurse, may also experience similar stages.

a The following situation consists of segments of interactions occurring over time between a nurse and a dying woman. In the situation a variety of different communication skills are used by the nurse to facilitate the client's progress through the dying process. Each communication skill has been italicized and numbered. Place the number of the examples in the space provided after each communication skill. A communication skill may be illustrated more than once; an example may illustrate more than one skill. The first one has been filled in to help you get started.

Communication skills

a. Clarifying _____   e. Giving reassurance _____

b. Encouraging _____   f. Reflecting _____

c. Exloring _____   g. Seeking information __1__

d. Focusing _____   h. Suggesting _____

i. Understanding _____

SITUATION

Stage One: Denial

(After entering the client's room and greeting her, the nurse asks:)

1. N *"Have you seen your doctor today, Helen?"*
    C "Yes, Martha. He just left."
2. N *"And?"*
    C "Oh, he said something about a tumor. But I don't understand all that technical talk. It's too much for my feeble brain." (Laughingly.)
3. N *"Are there any questions I can try and answer for you?"*
    C "No. That's OK. You know what they say. What you don't know can't hurt you."
4. N *"You don't want to talk about it?"*
    C "Not yet. Why borrow trouble? Anyway, the doctor said I am going to have more tests. No sense worrying until all the results are in."
5. N *"It sounds a little like you are worrying now."*
    C "A little bit. But I'm trying to put those fears out of my head. But it's hard, being in the hospital, surrounded by the sounds and smells of sick people. I keep telling myself that it's happening to them, not me."
6. N *"Do you want to talk about those fears?"*
    C "No, Martha. I don't think so. Let's wait and see what happens. There will be lots of time for talking later. And, maybe if I'm lucky there will be nothing to talk about."
7. N *"I just want you to know that I'm here for you when you need me. I'll be happy to listen when you feel like talking."*
    C "Thank you, Martha." (Whispering.) "I'll remember that. I may need you." (Briskly, loudly.) "Now, let's talk about something else. Let me tell you about my daughter, Janie."

Stage Two: Anger

(The nurse enters the client's room and greets her.)

8. N *"How are you today, Helen?"*
    C "Terrible!" (The client sits stiffly in bed, a frown on her face, gripping the bed clothes tightly.)
9. N *"What's the matter?"*
    C "Where have you been? You should have been here an hour ago."
10. N *"I don't understand. What has happened to make you so upset?"*
    C "I was climbing the walls!"

11. **N** *"You are saying you were in pain?"*

    C "Pain's not the word for it. Why do I have to suffer so? And I was all alone. No one cares what happens to me."

12. **N** *"You sound pretty angry, Helen."*

    C "You bet I'm angry."

13. **N** *"Perhaps you'd like to tell me about it."*

    C "Well, I finally got my medication. The nurse gave it to me early. But what I had to go through to get it! I can take anything except the pain."

14. **N** *"There is no need for you to hurt so. I'll speak with your doctor about shortening the time between your doses. Now, let me rub your back and help ease up those tense muscles. Then we can talk more if you like."*

Stage Three: Bargaining

(When the nurse enters the client's room, the client initiates the conversation.)

    C "Hi, Martha. It's Janie's birthday Saturday."

15. **N** *"Really? She'll be 13, won't she?"*

    C "Yes. My baby is growing up."

16. **N** *"You have two boys besides Janie, don't you?"*

    C "Twin boys. They were 15 when she was born. They are grown and on their own now. I'm not worried about them."

17. **N** *"But you're worried about Janie?"*

    C "She's now a teenager. That's such a difficult time these days. She's just beginning to be interested in boys. I wish I could be home to talk with her. We were just starting to have some good mother-daughter talks when I got sick and had to come to the hospital. I miss them . . . and her." The client continues, "We talk on the phone some, but it's not the same. And she visits. But there is no real privacy here. And even if there was, it wouldn't be the same. She needs a mother's love and constant guidance. I don't want to let her down."

18. **N** *"Let her down?"*

    C "Yes. I wish I could stay around long enough to see that she gets a good education and a good start in life. I think I could rest easy if I saw her married to a good man . . . I've not always been the most cooperative patient. Sometimes I've given the nurses a hard time. I figure that if I do everything I'm told and try to be a good patient, I'll help my chances of getting better. Oh, I don't mean a miracle or anything like that. Just well enough to see Janie grown up and on her own." (Silence.)

19. **N** *"Go on."*

20. **N** *"You don't think you've been a cooperative patient?"*

Stage Four: Depression

(The nurse enters the client's room and finds Helen lying in the dark, bed curtains partly drawn. An untouched dinner tray is on the overbed table. Martha checks to see that Helen is awake and then offers to sit with her for a while.)

21. **N** *"You haven't eaten your supper . . . and you've been crying."* (Silence.)

22. **N** *"Perhaps it would help to talk about what you are feeling."*

    C "What's the use of talking? It won't change anything."

23. **N** *"You sound pretty down tonight."*

    C "There's no fight left in me anymore. This is the beginning of the end."

24. **N** *"That's what you've been afraid of all along?"*

    C "Yes. But I couldn't admit it. It's time I faced the truth."

25. **N** *"Go on Helen."*

    C "I did feel better for a bit. The treatments seemed to be helping, and I thought I had it licked. But I'm not better, not really. I'll never get better." (Crying.)

(Silence. The nurse reaches over and takes Helen's hand. The client grips it tightly.)

26. **N** *"It must be frightening for you to be thinking these thoughts. You tried so hard to push them aside."*

    C "It's no use. I'm getting weaker. Even little things I used to do for myself, like comb my hair, are an effort. I'm slipping every day. There is nothing left to live for." (Silence.)

    C "The past keeps going through my mind. I remember all the things my husband and I did before he died. And then I think of all the things I wanted to do with my life but will never get to do. It makes me feel so sad."

27. **N** *"What things? Tell me about them."*

    C "Well, like raising Janie. There's so much I want to do with her, to tell her, to teach her. . . . At this rate I won't get to see her fourteenth birthday. . . . And I always wanted to paint. I planned to take art classes after Janie was grown and I had more time. You know, I had this fantasy that I would be another Grandma Moses in my old age. Old age! Ha! I won't have to worry about that. It's very depressing to look back on your life and feel so incomplete, to see so many loose ends."

28. **N** *"Have you given any thought as to how you might tie up some of those loose ends?"*

    C "Well, yes. But I don't know. Maybe it's silly."

29. **N** *"Silly?"*

    C "Yes. I thought about writing a diary or filling a notebook with some of the things I've been thinking and feeling. To share with Janie. Something to leave her when I'm gone. Is that a silly idea? My sister promised to care for her when I'm gone. In fact she's with her now. I know she's in good hands. I don't worry about that anymore. But I want her to have something of me. To remember me by."

30. **N** *"You'd like to write down some of your thoughts and feelings for Janie to read later, when she is older?"*

    C "That's right. There is so much I want to share with her." (Excitedly.) "Recollections of when she was a baby, of her father, of the things we did as a family. Also, I want her to know how much I loved her, how much pleasure she gave her father and me, about our hopes for her future. . . . What do you think? Is it silly?

31. **N** *"It sounds like a very loving thing to do."*

    C "I'd like to start right away. I don't have much time left. . . . You know, I feel better now. Would you open my bed curtains and turn on the light? Maybe I'll try some of that applesauce on my tray now."

32. **N** *"Let me get some hot water and I'll fix you a fresh cup of tea before I leave. And would you like me to bring you a notebook and a pen so you can start writing?"*

    C "Oh yes. That would be splendid."

33. **N** *"And, I was thinking . . . perhaps you would like some art paper and paints so you could try your hand at painting."*

    C "Do you think I could? Really?"

Stage Five: Acceptance

(The nurse enters the room and finds Helen sleeping. She sits down beside the bed and sometime later Helen rouses and sees Martha sitting nearby.)

    C "Oh, you're here, Martha. Have you been sitting there long?"

34. **N** *"No, just a few minutes. I thought I would look in on you and see how you were doing before I left for the day. Is there anything I can do for you?"*

    C "No, thank you. I'm all right. I've been napping a lot lately."

35. **N** *"How are you feeling?"*

    C "Pretty tired. I'm glad I've finished Janie's notebook. I don't think I would have the strength to write anymore. . . . And I've stopped painting too. But I got a lot done, didn't I?" (Pointing with obvious pride and pleasure to the numerous paintings on the walls of her room.) "That was a godsend. I enjoyed painting, but now I'm just content to lie here and look at them. . . . You know, if it hadn't been for you, I would never have fulfilled my dream to paint before I die. Would you like to have one of my pictures? It would please me if you would take one."

36. **N** *"I would like that too. Thank you. I'd enjoy having something you painted. . . . Are you comfortable?*
    C "Yes. The medications keep me free of pain. At this point, that's all I ask. But they do make me sleepy. It's an effort to keep my eyes open."
37. **N** *"It's OK. Close them. I'll be right here with you. I'll stay until you fall asleep and then I'll be back tomorrow."*
    C "Please hold my hand, Martha."

(The nurse takes Helen's hand and sits quietly with her. Before she leaves, Martha promises to give Janie the notebook after Helen dies. She also selects the painting she will keep. Helen died the next day. Martha was with her.)

b Complete the following exercises using the grid provided.

1. Describe the general characteristics of each stage of dying.
2. Refer to the previous situation and briefly describe behavioral responses observed in the client that illustrate each of the five stages of dying.

Stages of dying	Characteristics	Behaviors
1. Denial		
2. Anger		
3. Bargaining		
4. Depression		
5. Acceptance		

TEST ITEMS

1 Which one of the following is the *most* therapeutic nursing response to use with persons who are dealing with emotional reactions precipitated by a physical illness?

    a Reassuring them that they will feel better after a while.

    b Sympathizing with them over their situation.

    c Attending to their fears and concerns.

    d Giving them complete information about their condition.

2 The experience of dehumanization can *best* be avoided by which one of the following measures?

    a Treating the client at home rather than in the hospital.

    b Allowing the client unlimited visiting hours.

    c Introducing the client to persons with similar problems.

    d Listening to and answering the client's questions.

3 Self-help groups are helpful because the affected individual is:

    a Allowed to replace medical supervision with peer supervision.

    b Encouraged to relate to others with similar problems rather than relate to nonaffected individuals.

    c Helped to decrease dependency on nurses, family members, and close friends.

    d Provided with emotional support and understanding from persons who share the same health problem.

4 A young diabetic client who neglected a serious infection in his leg had to have a below-the-knee amputation. After surgery he refused to eat or talk with anyone. Which of the following is the *most* probable explanation of his behavior?

    a Guilt for neglecting to care for himself.

    b Grief for loss of a body part.

    c Fear that he might lose his other leg.

    d Anger at the surgeon who removed his leg.

5 Emotional reactions precipitated by the loss of a body part are usually related to:

    a Changed perception of self.

    b Concern over disposal of the body part.

    c Inability to cope with feelings of guilt.

    d Unconscious feelings associated with punishment.

6 Disfiguring and mutilating-type surgery is especially difficult for individuals to accept. Which one of the following is generally *least* traumatic?

    a Repair of a hare lip.   c Colostomy.

    b Radical mastectomy.   d Prostatectomy.

7 Immediately following cardiac surgery the client is *most* likely to need help with which one of the following?

   a Guilt feelings.   c Sexual urges.

   b Dependency conflicts.   d Body image.

8 Women who give birth to premature infants or babies born with congenital imperfections generally respond by:

   a Expressing feelings of guilt.

   b Rejecting the infant.

   c Questioning their adequacy as women.

   d All of the above.

9 When a client who has been living in fear of AIDS finally has the diagnosis confirmed, he or she will often respond initially with feelings of:

   a Denial.   c Relief.

   b Anger.   d Depression.

10 When giving nursing care to a client with AIDS the nurse should always:

   a Utilize strict isolation precautions.

   b Limit the use of touch.

   c Supervise visits by family and friends.

   d Respond with sensitivity and respect.

11 Which one of the following nursing diagnoses using the ANA format is *most* specific to a client in the late stages of AIDS?

   a Altered Sleep/Arousal Patterns R/T fear of dying (1.4.2).

   b Altered Thought Process R/T viral invasion of the CNS (2.6.2).

   c Suicide Attempt R/T feelings of despair (5.3.2.9).

   d Loneliness R/T rejection by family and friends (8.1.2.3).

12 According to Elisabeth Kübler-Ross, the initial response to impending death is:

   a Anger.   c Depression.

   b Bargaining.   d Denial.

13 Although all of the following manifestations may be present, which one is *least likely* to be observed in a client during the depression stage of dying?

   a Sad affect.   c Sarcasm.

   b Cooperative behavior.   d Silence.

14 Acceptance, the final stage of dying, is mostly characterized by feelings of:

   a Relief.   c Sadness.

   b Peacefulness.   d Regret.

15 To be truly effective in helping a dying person the nurse must *first*:

   a Identify the five stages of dying.

   b Profess strong religious convictions.

   c Develop greater self-awareness.

   d Accept the inevitability of death.

Section four word games and section exercises

1 Matching

a Historical perspective

DIRECTIONS: Listed below are the names of ten persons who have contributed significantly to the fields of psychiatry and psychiatric-mental health nursing. Also listed are their contributions. Match the person with their contribution by placing the number of the contribution in the space provided by the contributor. The first one has been filled in to help you get started.

Contributions	Contributors
1. Identified the role of anxiety in one's unconscious life.	___ Alexander
2. Pioneer in thanatology.	___ Alzheimer
3. Introduced, with Bini, the use of electroconvulsive therapy.	___ Bleuler
4. Authority in the treatment of individuals with borderline personality disorder.	___ Cerletti
5. Introduced the term "schizophrenia."	_1_ Freud
6. German neurologist who treated presenile dementia.	___ Kernberg
7. Originator of the *Fight or Flight Theory*.	___ Krapelin
8. Developed insulin shock therapy.	___ Kübler-Ross
9. ". . . emptiness and hopelessness are all a measure of the basic loneliness and anxiety of our time."	___ Moustakos
10. One of the first to recognize the cyclical nature of manic-depressive psychosis.	___ Sakel

b Psychotropic medications

DIRECTIONS: Listed below and on p. 231 are the trade or brand names of thirty-five psychotropic medications. Fill in the grid, matching the trade name with the appropriate generic name. In several instances there may be more than one trade medication for a generic name, such as in the case of Lithium. The trade names of Lithium Carbonate, Lithane, Lithonate, and Eskalith have been filled in to help you get started.

Trade or Brand Names

ADAPIN	✔ LITHIUM CARBONATE	PAMELOR	STELAZINE
ATIVAN	✔ LITHONATE	PARNATE	TARACTAN
AVENTYL	LOXITANE	PAXIPAM	THORAZINE
CENTRAX	MARPLAN	PERTOFRANE	TOFRANIL
ELAVIL	MELLARIL	PROLIXIN	TRANXENE
✔ ESKALITH	MOBAN	QUIDE	TRILAFON
HALDOL	NARDIL	SERAX	VALIUM
LIBRIUM	NAVANE	SERENTIL	XANAX
✔ LITHANE	NORPRAMIN	SINEQUAN	

	Chemical classification	Trade name	Generic name
Antipsychotic	Phenothiazine derivative: Aliphatic subgroup	1. _____	Chlorpromazine
	Phenothiazine derivatives: Piperidine subgroup	2. _____	Thioridazine
		3. _____	Piperacetazine
		4. _____	Mesoridazine
	Phenothiazine derivatives: Piperazine subgroup	5. _____	Fluphenazine
		6. _____	Perphenazine
		7. _____	Trifluoperazine
	Butyrophenone derivative	8. _____	Haloperidol
	Thioxanthene derivatives	9. _____	Chlorprothixene
		10. _____	Thiothixene
	Dihydroindolone derivative	11. _____	Molindone
	Dibenzoxazepine derivative	12. _____	Loxapine succinate

	Chemical classification	Trade name	Generic name
Antidepressant	Tricyclics	13. _____	Imipramine
		14. _____	Amitriptyline
		15. _____	Desipramine
		16. _____	Nortriptyline
		17. _____	
		18. _____	Doxepin
		19. _____	
		20. _____	
	Monoamine oxidase inhibitors	21. _____	Isocarboxazid
		22. _____	Phenelzine sulfate
		23. _____	Tranylcypromine
Antimanic	Lithium	24. Lithium Carbonate	Lithium carbonate
		25. Eskalith	
		26. Lithane	
		27. Lithonate	
Anxiolytic	Benzodiazepine group	28. _____	Diazepam
		29. _____	Alprazolam
		30. _____	Chlordiazepoxide
		31. _____	Clorazepate dipotassium
		32. _____	Halazepam
		33. _____	Lorazepam
		34. _____	Oxazepam
		35. _____	Prazepam

2 Crosshatch

DIRECTIONS: Fit the eighty-two words listed on p. 232 into the proper boxes. The words read left to right or top to bottom, one letter per box. CON-SUMERS has been entered to give you a starting point. (Solution appears in the Appendix.)

3 letters
DSM
ECT
EGO
FAT
LAW
NOS
SHY

4 Letters
ACID
AIDS
BODY
CARE
FEAR
HATE
MOOD
PLAN
TOOL

5 letters
ACUTE
ANGER
BINGE
DYING
FIGHT
GAINS
MANIC
NEEDS
NOTME
SHOCK

6 letters
AFFECT
ATAXIA
AUTISM
CLIENT
COPING
CRISIS
DENIAL
ENERGY
FLIGHT
HEROIN
LISTEN
OPIATE
PHOBIA
SENILE
SORROW

7 letters
BIPOLAR
BULIMIA
COCAINE
DESPAIR
DEVIANT
ELATION
EMPATHY
LITHIUM
MIDLIFE
ORGANIC
SUBTYPE
SUICIDE
SYMPTOM
TRUANCY

8 letters
ANOREXIA
CONFLICT
DELUSION
HOLISTIC
HYSTERIA
NEUROTIC
PARANOID

9 letters
ALOOFNESS
BODY IMAGE
CATATONIC
CONFUSION
CONSUMERS
PSYCHOSIS
SOCIOPATH
TOLERANCE
TREATMENT

10 letters
ACCEPTANCE
COMPULSION
CONVERSION
DERAILMENT
EVALUATION
FLAT AFFECT
LIFE REVIEW
NEGATIVISM
WITHDRAWAL

11 letters
INTERACTION
THANATOLOGY

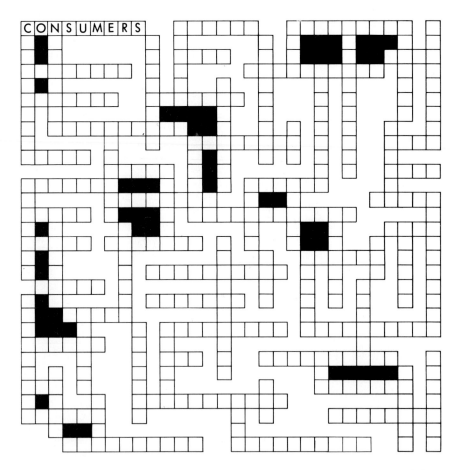

3 Quote-a-crostic

DIRECTIONS: Using cues on the left, fill in the words in the list on the right. Transfer each letter in the word list to the corresponding numbered square in the puzzle grid. Shaded squares in the grid represent the end of a word. Work back and forth between grid and word list until both are completed. (Note the letters and consecutive numbers that have been entered in the grid to help in location of words.) The completed grid will be a quotation relevant to Section IV of the text. The source of the quote and its author are spelled out in the boxed-in letters in the word list. One word in the list has been filled in to help you get started. (Solution appears in the Appendix.)

Cues

Word list

A Subjective cue to pathology

___ ___ ___ | ___ | ___ ___ ___
137 116 71 8 106 124 97

B Victorian term for unexplained fatigue and weakness

___ ___ ___ ___ | ___ | ___ ___ ___
51 22 166 113 155 162 129 75

C Significant other

___ ___ ___ ___ ___ | ___ |
108 7 94 107 176 56

D DSM-III-R 302.70 Sexual _____ NOS

___ ___ | ___ | ___ ___ ___ ___ ___ ___ ___ ___
93 199 98 70 150 32 140 50 84 118 171

E Seclusion (two words)

___ ___ ___ ___ ___   ___ | ___ | ___ ___
149 119 48 55 179   115 167 69 79

F Moustakos: ". . . emptiness and hopelessness are all a measure of the basic _____ and anxiety of our time."

___ ___ | ___ | ___ ___ ___ ___ ___ ___ ___
90 58 190 39 100 184 159 130 123 205

G "A person who talks about suicide never attempts suicide."

___ ___ ___ | ___ |
60 78 41 13

H Nonspecific response to stress

___ ___ ___ ___ ___ ___ ___ ___ | ___ | ___
61 24 30 54 33 45 4 91 141 148

I Doctors' medication instructions

| ___ | ___ ___ ___ ___ ___
2 59 161 72 177 82

J Disorder related to lack of light during winter months (abb.)

___ ___ | ___ |
86 138 46

K NANDA: 7.3.2

___ ___ ___ ___ ___ | ___ | ___ ___ ___ ___ ___ ___ ___
29 87 104 20 156 128 10 195 198 80 187 174 117

L Addicted to heroin (slang)

___ ___ ___ ___ | ___ | ___
142 202 27 40 99 172

M Symptom of despair

S | O | B S
132 143 89 157

233

N Flat, blunt, or inappropriate
___ ___ ___ ___ ___ ___
178 131 28 111 200 64

O Grief
___ ___ ___ ___ ___ ___ ___ ___ ___ ___ ___
12 6 146 96 81 19 173 1 122 112 74

P ANA: 7.1.1.1 _____ _____ Deficit (two words)
___ ___ ___ ___ ___   ___ ___ ___ ___ ___ ___
57 152 133 180 160   44 194 63 163 110 35

Q Nurses' written records
___ ___ ___ ___ ___
73 14 145 127 203

R Disorganized, paranoid, undifferentiated, catatonic, or residual
___ ___ ___ ___ ___ ___ ___ ___ ___ ___ ___ ___ ___
68 85 95 204 154 193 175 34 126 43 182 23 114

S Characteristic of children with attention deficits
___ ___ ___ ___ ___ ___ ___ ___ ___ ___ ___
201 36 66 196 120 147 134 16 170 188 52

T Human response pattern (two words)
___ ___ ___ ___ ___ ___ ___ ___ ___ ___ ___ ___ ___
5 135 65 103 153 109 185 42 77 31 121 11 144
___ ___ ___ ___ ___ ___ ___ ___ ___
197 15 181 191 47 3 165 18 37

U Psychiatric _____ _____ nursing (two words)
___ ___ ___ ___ ___ ___   ___ ___ ___ ___ ___ ___
168 67 92 49 158 186   17 102 26 76 83 192

V Reminiscence (two words)
___ ___ ___ ___   ___ ___ ___ ___ ___ ___
9 105 125 38   88 25 101 151 169 183

W Physical problem often associated with onset of bronchial asthma
___ ___ ___ ___ ___ ___ ___
136 139 62 189 21 164 53

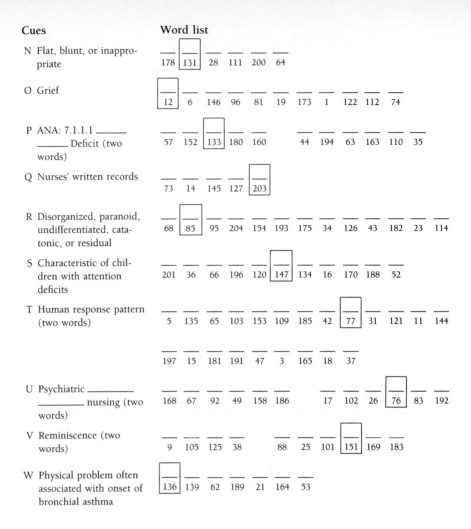

1 O	2 I	3 T	4 H	■	5 T	6 O	7 C	8 A	9 V	10 K	■	11 T	12 O	13 G	14 Q	15 T	■	16 S	17 U	18 T	■	19 O	20 K
21 W	22 B	■	23 R	24 H	25 V	26 U	■	27 L	28 N	■	29 K	30 H	31 T	32 D	■	33 H	34 R	35 P	36 S	■	37 T	38 V	39 F
40 L	■	41 G	42 T	■	43 R	44 P	45 H	46 J	47 T	■	48 E	49 U	■	50 D	51 B	52 S	53 W	■	54 H	55 E	56 C	57 P	58 F
59 I	60 G	■	61 H	62 W	63 P	64 N	65 T	66 S	67 U	68 R	■	69 E	70 D	■	71 A	72 I	73 Q	74 O	75 B	76 U	■	77 T	78 G
79 E	80 K	81 O	82 I	83 U	84 D	85 R	86 J	■	87 K	88 V	■	89 M (B)	90 F	91 H	92 V	93 D	■	94 C	95 R	96 O	97 A	98 D	99 L
100 F	101 V	102 U	103 T	■	104 K	105 V	106 A	107 C	■	108 C	109 T	110 P	111 N	112 O	113 B	114 R	115 E	116 A	■	117 K	118 D	119 E	120 S	121 T
122 O	123 F	■	124 A	125 V	■	126 R	127 Q	128 K	129 B	130 F	131 N	■	132 M (S)	133 P	134 S	135 T	■	136 W	137 A	■	138 J	139 W	140 D	141 H
142 L	143 M (O)	144 T	■	145 Q	146 O	147 S	148 H	149 E	150 D	151 V	152 P	153 T	154 R	155 B	156 K	157 M (S)	■	158 U	159 F	160 P	■	161 I	162 B	163 P
164 W	165 T	■	166 B	167 E	168 U	169 V	■	170 S	171 D	■	172 L	173 O	174 K	175 R	176 C	177 I	■	178 N	179 E	180 P	181 T	182 R	■	183 V	184 F
185 T	186 U	■	187 K	188 S	189 W	190 F	■	191 T	192 U	193 R	194 P	195 K	196 S	■	197 T	198 K	199 D	200 N	201 S	202 L	203 Q	204 R	205 F

24 | Crisis theory and intervention

INTRODUCTION

In the course of day-to-day living many challenges, changes, and stresses threaten a person's equilibrium. Using problem-solving methods, coping measures, and defense mechanisms, one strives to maintain a healthy personality balance and continue to function effectively. When the usual methods of dealing with problems fail, anxiety increases, disorganization occurs, and crisis results. Helplessness is experienced and the individual is incapable of taking positive action to deal with the situation and is a candidate for crisis intervention.

"Crisis intervention is a subject of interest to all health professionals. It is a technique that is used successfully by persons with a variety of backgrounds to aid individuals and families in understanding and effectively coping with the intense emotions that characterize a crisis state."* The goal of intervention in a crisis state is to help solve immediate, seemingly insurmountable problems. Individuals in crisis are helped to face and eventually handle their problems within the framework of their support system, mobilizing coping and defense mechanisms to deal with the critical event. The goal of crisis intervention is based on the belief that persons in crisis possess strengths that have been temporarily overwhelmed. With timely, short-term intervention, persons in crisis are given the support necessary to solve their immediate problems. Ideally, they are helped to emerge from the experience stronger and more confident in their abilities to meet subsequent stresses in growth-promoting ways.

The exercises in this chapter are designed to help you review the phases and characteristics of a crisis state and identify nursing actions that can be taken to intervene therapeutically in a crisis state.

---

*From Taylor CM: Mereness' essentials of psychiatric nursing, ed 13, St Louis, 1990, The CV Mosby Co, chap 24.

1. To define crisis.
2. To differentiate between developmental and situational events that precipitate crisis states.
3. To list the general characteristics of a crisis state.
4. To link characteristic behavioral responses to the phases of crisis in which they are generally seen.
5. To review communication skills used to intervene therapeutically with the individual in crisis.
6. To reflect on one's ability to deal with stress.

EXERCISES

1 Define crisis:

2 Listed below are fifteen events that may precipitate a state of crisis. Read each one and determine whether it illustrates a developmental or situational crisis. Place a check in the box in the appropriate column. The first one has been filled in to help you get started.

Events	Crisis	
	Developmental	Situational
1. Birth of a new baby.	☑	☐
2. Retirement from a job.	☐	☐
3. Aging parent moves into nursing home.	☐	☐
4. Moving out-of-state.	☐	☐
5. Death of an aging parent.	☐	☐
6. Adolescent has sexual intercourse for first time.	☐	☐
7. Loss of a limb in an accident.	☐	☐
8. Child marries and leaves home.	☐	☐
9. Promotion at work.	☐	☐
10. Vacation or leisure.	☐	☐
11. Stillbirth.	☐	☐
12. Failure to graduate with one's class.	☐	☐
13. Loss of one's home by fire.	☐	☐
14. Onset of menopausal symptoms.	☐	☐
15. Mother has a radical mastectomy.	☐	☐

3 List below four *general* characteristics of a crisis state:

a _____

b _____

c _____

d _____

4 A crisis state tends to follow a predictable and sequential pattern of phases. Characteristically, the first response to an event that precipitates a crisis is *denial*. The individual unconsciously refuses to acknowledge the traumatic event. This phase, however, leads rather quickly into the phase of *increased tension* in which the person attempts to ward off increasing amounts of anxiety with hyperactivity or psychomotor retardation. The phase of *disorganization* follows, and at this time the individual is no longer able to function, becomes preoccupied with the precipitating event, and is generally overwhelmed with anxiety. The next phase is one of several phases that reflect the individual's attempts to *reorganize*. Coping measures are used to deal with the crisis. If these measures fail, the individual may experience the phase characterized by an attempt to *escape the problem*. It is at this time that the individual in crisis blames others for the problem or situation. Another method used to escape the problem is to consciously pretend it does not exist. These measures are rarely successful, and the individual again attempts to reorganize. The phase at this time is called *local reorganization* and is followed by the phase of *general reorganization*. The three phases of reorganization, although occurring at different times during the crisis state, share similar behavioral manifestations and for the purposes of this exercise are grouped together. Listed below and on p. 238 are twelve behavioral examples that characterize these phases of a crisis state. Identify which behavior reflects which phase and place a check in the box in the appropriate column. The first one has been filled in to help you get started.

	Phases of crisis				
Behavioral examples	Denial	Increased tension	Disorganization	Reorganization	Escape the problem
1. Arthur refused to take the storm warnings seriously, and his home was destroyed.	☑	☐	☐	☐	☐
2. After days of inactivity in which he had been unable to function, Lee mobilized himself and resumed swimming at the club.	☐	☐	☐	☐	☐
3. Francis became overwhelmed with anxiety and thought she was "losing her mind" after her infant son died of crib death.	☐	☐	☐	☐	☐
4. Gregory ignored his financial advisors, subsequently lost millions of dollars, and then blamed them for his loss.	☐	☐	☐	☐	☐
5. Following the death of a loved one, Lincoln insisted on making all the funeral arrangements himself.	☐	☐	☐	☐	☐
6. Mary could not face the truth and returned to work after she was fired.	☐	☐	☐	☐	☐
7. Zoe would not acknowledge the fact that she had less than 6 months to live and enrolled in law school.	☐	☐	☐	☐	☐

Continued.

Behavioral examples	Denial	Increased tension	Disorganization	Reorganization	Escape the problem
			Phases of crisis		
8. Following the airplane crash that killed his entire family, Jack became very preoccupied with the accident and could talk about nothing else.	☐	☐	☐	☐	☐
9. With great effort to focus on things other than her recent loss, Alma was finally able to resume her everyday activities.	☐	☐	☐	☐	☐
10. Robinson failed to install a smoke detector in his apartment and when it was destroyed by fire, he blamed his landlord.	☐	☐	☐	☐	☐
11. Stella was unable to function and experienced tremendous anxiety after being raped at knife point.	☐	☐	☐	☐	☐
12. When Maggie learned her unmarried teenage daughter was pregnant, she engaged in accelerated housecleaning.	☐	☐	☐	☐	☐

5 Because persons in crisis are not always aware that they are in crisis and respond with feelings of helplessness and puzzlement, the nurse must often use a very direct, straightforward approach when intervening therapeutically in a crisis state. Passive, nondirective interviewing techniques have limited use in the initial contacts with the client.

Within the framework of the nursing process, the nurse uses a variety of communication skills to interact therapeutically with the individual in crisis. The initial phase of assessment involves collecting data, reviewing the events leading up to the crisis, identifying the event that most probably precipitated the crisis, helping identify the protagonists in the crisis, and helping the client focus on feelings and thoughts relevant to the crisis. The nurse directs the interview so that the client is helped to express the gamut of feelings being experienced: anxiety, fear, pain, loss, anger, depression, helplessness, and frustration. Once this is done, the nurse and the person in crisis can develop a plan of action for coping with the critical situation. This includes helping the client identify resources to reduce the feelings of isolation so often experienced. As the person in crisis feels support, defenses and coping measures are mobilized to deal with the situation.

In the following situation Mary Edwards, a client in crisis, has been taken to the emergency room of the local hospital where she is interviewed by a nurse skilled in crisis intervention. A variety of therapeutic skills are illustrated. They have been numbered and italicized. Place the number of the examples in the space provided after each communication skill. A communication skill may be illustrated more than once; an example may illustrate more than one skill. The first one has been filled in to help you get started.

Communication skills

a Clarifying _____   f Reflecting _____

b Direct questioning _____   g Refocusing _____

c Encouraging _____   h Seeking information _____

d Focusing _1_____   i Suggesting _____

e Giving reassurance _____   j Understanding _____

SITUATION

N   "My name is Susan Lamb. I am a nurse. Your name is Mary Edwards. I would like to help you, Mary."

C   (Crying.)

1. **N**   *"Let's talk about what you are feeling."*

   C   (Mary continues to cry.)

2. **N**   *"I understand that you live in a house in the beach area that was hardest hit by the hurricane."*

   C   (Nodding.)

3. **N**   *"How long have you lived there?"*

   C   "Thirty years."

4. **N**   *"That's a long time. You must have a lot of memories invested in that house."*

   C   "We had a lot of good times there. Oh, what am I going to do? I can't go on. There is no use in going on." (Mary continues to cry.)

5. **N**   *"It sounds like you are feeling terribly discouraged right now."*

   C   "I don't know what I am going to do. How am I going to face my husband? (Crying and wringing her hands.)

6. **N**   *"Where is your husband now?"*

   C   "John is here, upstairs on the surgical ward. He had an operation a few days ago. Oh John, John. . . . If he hadn't gone to the hospital this would never have happened. He left me all alone."

7. **N**   *"Do you have any children, Mary?"*

   C   "Two. They are grown and on their own. I was pregnant with a third child 6 years ago, but I miscarried. That was terrible." (Mary resumes crying.)

8. **N**   *"You were telling me about your children. Your two grown children."* (Mary tells the nurse about Emma Lou, age 26, and John, Jr., age 24, who are married and living out-of-state. She begins to cry again as she recalls them and the life they all shared in the destroyed home. The nurse reaches over and takes Mary's hand, and the client grips it tightly.)

9. **N**   *"I'm here for you. I'm going to help you through this time."*

   C   (Nodding.)

10. **N**   *"Go on. Tell me more."*

    C   "It's the first time I've been alone in my life. Before John, I had my parents. When they died, he was there to help me through it. When the children left home, John and I faced it together. But now. . . . " (Crying.)

11. **N**   *"Now you feel as if there is no one you can turn to?"*

    C   "He shouldn't have left me. He knows this is the hurricane season. He wanted me to do everything. To take care of the house. What do I know of such things? He has always done it." (Mary releases the nurse's hand and clenches her fists.)

12. **N**   *"You sound pretty angry with your husband."*

    C   "He's had that hernia for years. Why did he pick this time to go to the hospital?"

13. **N** *"Do you think he could have waited and had the operation later?"*

C "I guess not. The doctor said it was serious. But it's not fair. We worked hard all our lives. What did we do to deserve this? Oh, what am I going to tell John? What is he going to say?"

14. **N** *"What do you think he will say?"*

C "I don't know. I don't know. I'm afraid to face him."

15. **N** *"If it would help, I'll be glad to go upstairs with you when you go to see John."*

C "Oh yes. I think that would help."

16. **N** *"You both have reason to be upset. You've had your home destroyed."*

C "Thirty years down the drain."

17. **N** *"Are you talking about your home or your life?"*

C "My life, I guess." (The nurse waits while Mary cries briefly.)

C "I'm sorry. I can't stop crying. Every time I think about it I feel sort of panicky."

18. **N** *"That must be frightening for you."*

C (Nodding.)
(Silence.)

19. **N** *"Are you saying you have lost everything?"*

C "I guess so. But I really haven't lost everything, have I? I still have John. We are alive. Our children are safe. We have each other. We can start over."

20. **N** *"You can start over."*

21. **N** *"What do you need to do first?"*
(Client takes a deep breath and then lets it all out.)

C "I have to talk to John. But what am I going to say to him?"

22. **N** *"Let's think about that. Perhaps it would help for you to think through what you want to say to him."*

C "It's going to be hard to face him."

23. **N** *"Do you mean he will be angry with you?"*

C "Oh, no. I don't think so. He's probably going to be angry with himself and blame himself for not being there when I needed him. Oh no. He's a very special person. He's always been very understanding and supportive. I've always been able to count on him."

24. **N** *"You might feel better when you share your feelings with your husband."*

C "Yes, I believe I will."

25. **N** "All right. *So the first thing you are going to do is talk with John."*

26. **N** *"What about your son and daughter?"*

C "The children. I must let them know we are safe."

27. **N** *"Have you any other family you need to contact?"*

C "My sister Clara and her husband Carl. They must be frantic. They live on the other side of town. I must find out how they are."

28. **N** *"So you are going to contact your family."*

29. **N** *"What about where you are going to stay? Could you stay with your sister and brother-in-law for a while?"*

C "Yes. They have room. If they weren't affected by the storm (crying), I know I would have a place with them. The four of us are very close. John and Carl are business partners."

30. **N** *"That sounds like a good plan."*
(Silence.)

C "I wonder if we have disaster insurance?"

31. **N** *"Who is your insurance agent?"*

   C "I'm not sure. I'll have to ask John. You know I'm just realizing how dependent I am on John. I must find out more about our affairs so I can handle things better in the future."

32. **N** *"Yes? Go on."*

   C God forbid, but suppose something had happened to John. Suppose it was John I had lost, not just my house. I don't think I could manage." (Mary cries softly to herself.)

33. **N** *"That must be a frightening thing to realize. But you have time now to do something about that."*

34. **N** *"Review again what you are going to do."*

   C "First, I'm going to see John and talk with him. I want to get that over with."

35. **N** *"And then?"*

   C "Then I'll call Clara and Carl and the children."

36. **N** *"And you're going to check about your insurance agent."*
   (Client nods thoughtfully then says:)

   C "Five hours ago, when I saw what was left of our home, I didn't think there was anything left to live for. I wanted to curl up and die. I thought I was losing my mind."

37. **N** *"You had a terrible shock. It's not surprising you were feeling so overwhelmed."*

   C "Overwhelmed! That's it. I've never felt so overwhelmed and so alone in all my life. It was terrible. I still feel pretty shaky. I'm trying not to think about what has happened. I'm trying to focus on what I need to do now. But I hope I can remember everything I need to do."

38. **N** *"It wouldn't be too unusual for you to forget. You've been through a lot."*

39. **N** *"Perhaps it would help if you wrote down what you plan to do. Then you could share your plans with your husband when you see him."*

   C "Of course! A list. Why didn't I think of that myself? I always make lists. They keep me organized and I feel so accomplished when I cross off everything I've done."

40. **N** *"You seem to feel a little better now that you have a plan in mind."*

   C "As a matter of fact, I do feel somewhat better. A little while ago I thought my world was ended. Now I realize that only a small part of it is gone (crying), and I forgot about all that I have left to live for."

   N "I'm pleased you feel better. However, you have had a pretty tragic experience and you are bound to have some rough moments. I would like to see you again and find out how you are making out with your plans. Let's make an appointment for tomorrow. In the meantime here is my name and phone number in case you need anything before then. Also, I would like to know your sister's name, address, and phone number in case I need to reach you. Now let's work on your list and then you can go upstairs to visit your husband."

   C "Will you still go with me to see him?"

   N "Of course, I'd be glad to."

6 The ability to effectively deal with stress is influenced by several factors: personality strengths, membership in support groups, exposure to and handling of past crises, and expectations of others of how one will deal with crisis. In this exercise assess how well prepared you are to cope with stress by reflecting on the following questions. There are no right or wrong answers. The exercise is intended to open up some insights into your areas of strength as well as your areas of weakness, so that you may build on one and change the other. As a part of this exercise you may wish to share and discuss your perceptions with others with whom you feel comfortable.

a What do you see as your assets and wish to retain?

b What do you see as your limitations and would like to change?

c Who do you consider your closest friend(s)? How often do you contact them? How often do they contact you? Do you feel you can count on them for support?

d Who are your work/school associates? Do you feel you can count on them for support in work/school situations? Are you available to them if they need help? Do they know this?

e To what groups do you belong? How often are you in contact with these groups? What is your role in these groups? Do you experience satisfaction from membership in these groups? Are there other groups to which you would like to belong? Are your aspirations realistic?

f What was the most recent stressful event in your life? How did you handle it? Did you feel that you had to cope with it alone, or could you turn to others for help? Were you satisfied with your actions, with the outcome? Would you respond differently now? How? Why?

g Do you think other people see you as capable, somewhat capable, helpless, etc., in handling stressful occurrences? Do they look to you for help when they are having trouble coping? How do you feel about other people asking you for help?

TEST ITEMS

DIRECTIONS: Select the *best* response. (Answers appear in the Appendix.)

1 Which one of the following wars had the *greatest* impact on the evolution of crisis theory and intervention?
   a World War I.   c Korean War.
   b World War II.   d Vietnam War.

2 A person experiences a state of crisis when an event occurs that:
   a Evokes feelings of intense anxiety.
   b Is perceived as having traumatic proportions.
   c Fails to bring needed support from family members.
   d Is handled by coping measures.

3 There has been increasing interest in crisis intervention primarily because it is:
   a A short-term, reality-based treatment modality.
   b Less expensive than other forms of treatment.
   c Instrumental in preventing serious mental problems.
   d Providing job opportunities for health care workers.

4 The perception of a crisis as a "catalyst that disturbs old habits, evokes new responses, and becomes a major factor in charting new developments" is based on which one of the following outcomes of a crisis?

a Reintegration at a less healthy level of functioning.

b Reintegration at the same level of functioning.

c Reintegration at a higher level of functioning.

d None of the above.

5 The *unique* characteristic of a developmental crisis is:

    a Predictability.   **c** Anxiety.

    b Disequilibrium.   **d** Disorganization.

6 Which one of the following events might precipitate a *situational crisis?*

    a Mandatory draft registration.

    b Loss of a limb in an accident.

    c Death of an aging parent.

    d Retirement from a job.

7 Which one of the following events might precipitate a *developmental crisis?*

    a Birth of a new baby.

    b Retirement from a job following a coronary.

    c Death of a teenage son.

    d Change in life-style following a job promotion.

8 Which one of the following measures is *most* effective in helping a person cope with a developmental crisis?

    a Psychoanalysis.   **c** Psychotherapy.

    b Crisis intervention.   **d** Anticipatory guidance.

9 Basic to *all* behavioral responses to a crisis state is:

    a Anxiety.   **c** Depression.

    b Fear.   **d** Anger.

10 Failure to successfully deal with a crisis situation in 4 to 6 weeks usually results in repression of the experience and:

    a Free-floating anxiety.   **c** Pseudoresolution.

    b Increased tension.   **d** Denial.

11 During the phase of disorganization those in crisis:

    a Experience increased tension and hyperactivity.

    b Refuse to acknowledge they are in a state of crisis.

    c Become highly focused on the precipitating event.

    d Attempt to escape the problem by pretending it does not exist.

12 In the phase of crisis characterized by attempts to reorganize, the mechanism *most* used is:

    a Denial.   **c** Projection.

    b Suppression.   **d** Conversion.

13 After Marvin Young was fired because he was always late to work, he went through a period in which he blamed his mother, saying: "It's her fault I lost

my job. She never got me out of bed early enough." Marvin was experiencing which one of the following phases of a crisis state?

    a Attempts to escape.   c Disorganization.

    b Local reorganization.   d Denial.

14 In the initial stage of intervention in a crisis state, the nurse:

    a Assesses the situation.

    b Asks direct questions.

    c Identifies others involved in the problem.

    d All of the above.

15 In a crisis state the therapist can *most* effectively help persons cope with the situation by helping them identify:

    a The precipitating event.

    b Their available resources.

    c Feelings they are experiencing.

    d All of the above.

25 *Group theory and intervention*

INTRODUCTION

"A group is not a mere collection of individuals. Rather, a group is an identifiable system composed of three or more individuals who engage in certain tasks to achieve a common goal. Furthermore, to be a group the members must relate to each other, usually around the tasks and goals of the group."*

At the beginning of life, one automatically becomes a member of the family group. As the individual progresses through the stages of life, a multiplicity of group contacts are experienced: play and school groups, church affiliations, peer groups, and military, professional, business, community, political, recreational, and social associations. Because much of life takes place in group experiences, problems relating to other people are not only distressing but are also frequently incapacitating. Often interpersonal difficulties are the motivating forces behind a person's seeking professional help.

Nurses have an excellent opportunity to work with clients in a variety of different types of groups. An increasing number of professional nurses are acquiring the advanced educational preparation and skills needed to conduct formal therapy groups. In addition, nurses assume the role of socializing agents and facilitate relatedness and socialization among clients in both hospital and outpatient settings. For example, mealtime provides a good opportunity to promote social interaction between staff and clients. As role models, nurses demonstrate and help clients experience appropriate behaviors associated with food and eating. Similarly, activity groups can promote interaction and group relatedness, exposing clients to new and hopefully positive interpersonal experiences. Because experiences in one group contribute to a person's responsiveness in subsequent groups, the nurse can lay the groundwork for other positive group experiences and help an apparently unrelated individual become more socialized and less isolated.

My students generally work with long-term, severely withdrawn individuals. Part of their experience is to promote group interaction among their clients.

---

*From Taylor CM: Mereness' essentials of psychiatric nursing. ed 13, St Louis, 1990, The CV Mosby Co, chap 25.

245

Initially, because the clients are so resistive to relating, the groups tend to consist of more students than clients. Eventually, however, through the development of therapeutic nurse-client relationships in which the students become significant to their clients and through the use of a variety of tools—including food, games, music and song, rewards, and recognition—clients join and participate in the groups. In some cases the client may only participate during the final weeks of the experience. However, what has been found repeatedly is that the next group of students assigned to the service has a much easier task of involving the relatively stable group of clients in group activities. The clients require much less encouragement to participate, supporting the belief that one positive group experience will be instrumental in helping a client participate in other group experiences.

In addition to group work with clients, nurses often participate in meetings with other health care workers. In such groups the health care team engages in a variety of tasks, such as determining clients' needs, planning and evaluating client care, administering agency policies, and engaging in self-assessment. An understanding of the dynamics of group functioning and group process is a useful tool in making group activities at all levels more interesting and more effective. The exercises in this chapter are designed to help you increase your understanding of the nature of group experiences in general and therapeutic groups in particular.

OBJECTIVES

1. To identify the qualities that characterize most groups.
2. To analyze a hypothetical group interaction in terms of the roles assumed by the members.
3. To identify the characteristics of the four phases of group development.
4. To differentiate between formal therapy groups and socialization groups.

EXERCISES

1 Although groups differ in some respects, they tend to share certain characteristic qualities. In the following exercise are listed eight descriptive statements and eight characteristics about groups. Match each statement to the characteristic it describes by placing the number of the descriptive statement in the space provided by the characteristic.

Descriptive statements	Characteristics
1. A group is not just a collection of individuals but rather is an association of three or more people who meet to carry out a common task.	___ Attractiveness
2. In large groups members tend to break off into smaller groups.	___ Goals
3. All groups have a purpose for existing, and when the objectives are achieved, the group either identifies new ones or disbands.	___ Identity
4. Group members assume characteristic patterns of behavior that have either a content or a process orientation.	___ Membership
5. Groups establish rules by which they function.	___ Norms
6. Each group has a certain uniqueness based on size, goals, and membership.	___ Phases
7. Different groups have more appeal than others, based on membership, goals, and norms.	___ Roles
8. All groups progress through predictable stages of development.	___ Subgroups

2 The roles assumed by members of a group as suggested by Robert Bales are identified in the text and are in most cases self-descriptive. Eight group roles are listed in this exercise. Read the following situation involving members of a community group and identify the role assumed by each member of the group. In the space provided by each role write in the name of the member assuming that role. The group role of aggressor has been filled in to help you get started.

Group roles

a Aggressor _____Jason_____   e Information giver _____

b Blocker _____   f Information seeker _____

c Coordinator _____   g Orienter _____

d Harmonizer _____   h Recorder _____

SITUATION

Kirby	"We need to get started. Tina could not make tonight's meeting and asked that I chair the meeting in her absence."
Jason	"That's a mistake. I'm the most qualified person to do the job. I've had lots of experience leading groups."
Paula	"Maybe you can lead the meeting next time, Jason. This time Tina asked Kirby and sent him her agenda."
Carol	"I missed the last meeting. Could someone please bring me up to date on what happened last week?"
Tom	"Sure. We found we needed more information before we could reach a decision. Rob volunteered to check with the town council and report back to us. We agreed to table all decisions until we heard his report."
Kirby	"Thanks Tom. That about sums it up and gives us a good place to start. How about it, Rob? Tina had you first on the agenda. Are you ready to give us your report?"
Rob	"Yes. I made copies of some data and I'll distribute them to everyone."
Kirby	"Good. While Rob is doing that. . . . Let's see. . . . Arthur, I believe it's your turn to take minutes. OK?"
Arthur	Nods in agreement and gets out paper to write on.
Helen	"Why are we wasting time? There's no use in any of this. We've been through this a hundred times and nothing ever changes."
Jason	"I agree with Helen. Now I think we should proceed by. . . ."
Paula	"Come on you two. Let's hear Rob's report. Then we can decide our course of action."
Kirby	"OK everyone? All right Rob, you're on."
Rob	"Well, as you know I was to speak to the town council Monday. This is what I found out. If you look at the handout I gave you. . . . "

3 Every therapy group progresses through four developmental phases: preaffiliation, experiencing intragroup conflict, working or intimacy and differentiation, and termination. Listed on p. 248 are fifteen group goals, leader responsibilities, and member behaviors that are characteristic of different phases of a group's life. Differentiate among them by placing a check in the box in the appropriate column. The first one has been filled in to help you get started.

Characteristics	Phases			
	Preaffiliation	Intragroup conflict	Working	Termination
1. Members are cautious about developing relationships with each other.	☑	☐	☐	☐
2. Members share feelings of rejection, loss, and abandonment.	☐	☐	☐	☐
3. Leader accepts and supports power-control responses within the group.	☐	☐	☐	☐
4. Leader helps members think and work through problems.	☐	☐	☐	☐
5. Goal is to establish explicit norms to govern group functioning.	☐	☐	☐	☐
6. Members are highly cohesive and respond positively to suggestions made by fellow members.	☐	☐	☐	☐
7. Goal is to help members examine and alter behavioral patterns.	☐	☐	☐	☐
8. Leader orients members to the group process, to self, and to each other.	☐	☐	☐	☐
9. Members may withdraw and eventually drop out of the group.	☐	☐	☐	☐
10. Goal is to apply what has been learned in the group to other situations.	☐	☐	☐	☐
11. Leader encourages members to express feelings of loss.	☐	☐	☐	☐
12. Leader provides structure to the group and protects members from revealing themselves prematurely.	☐	☐	☐	☐
13. Members are strangers and distrustful of the leader and each other.	☐	☐	☐	☐
14. Members communicate readily, sharing and experiencing close feelings with each other.	☐	☐	☐	☐
15. Group sessions may seem unproductive due to alternating apathy and competition among the members.	☐	☐	☐	☐

4 Listed below are fifteen characteristics of formal therapy and socialization groups. Differentiate between them by placing a check in the box in the appropriate column. The first one has been filled in to help you get started.

Characteristics	Groups	
	Therapy	Socialization
1. Group size is generally limited to 6 to 10 people.	☑	☐
2. Attendance is variable, depending on the state of the individual at the time of the meeting.	☐	☐
3. Task-oriented activities are the major focus.	☐	☐
4. The ability to verbalize effectively is usually a criterion for membership.	☐	☐
5. Membership is relatively stable.	☐	☐
6. The development of trust is crucial to growth-promoting relationships.	☐	☐
7. Members are helped to deal more effectively with stress.	☐	☐
8. Beginning efforts at communication with others are encouraged.	☐	☐
9. Privacy and a quiet place to meet are essential.	☐	☐
10. A degree of ego strength is appropriate for membership.	☐	☐
11. Members are stimulated to take an interest in reality and in their surroundings.	☐	☐
12. Remotivation techniques are utilized.	☐	☐
13. Encourage the expression of feelings, ideas, and concerns.	☐	☐
14. Provide tangible rewards for participation.	☐	☐
15. Awareness of members' interests and hobbies provides a focus for activities.	☐	☐

DIRECTIONS: Select the *best* response. (Answers appear in the Appendix.)

1 Historically, group therapy was first used with which one of the following groups of clients?
   a Persons with tuberculosis.
   b Veterans suffering from "shell shock."
   c Psychotic individuals.
   d Persons with anxiety disorders.

2 Group therapy has been found to be the treatment of choice for many individuals because it:
   a Provides support to members when they realize that there are others with similar problems.
   b Simulates the family, a natural group, and allows them to work out familial difficulties.
   c Has been found to be a more efficient use of psychiatric personnel.
   d All of the above.

3 What would be the *least* number of members to constitute a group?
   a Two.   c Five.
   b Three.   d Ten.

4 Which one of the following roles assumed by group members is essentially a task- or content-oriented role?
   a Energizer.   c Observer.
   b Compromiser.   d Harmonizer.

5 Which one of the following roles assumed by group members is considered a group maintenance role?
   a Orienter.   c Recorder.
   b Elaborator.   d Encourager.

6 Which one of the following is the *best* example of a group norm?
   a Members assume a variety of task and/or group maintenance roles.
   b Members assemble weekly in a building where smoking is prohibited.
   c Members decide that everyone will address each other by first names.
   d Members modify their behavior to adapt to the group's uniqueness.

7 The membership of a "balanced" therapy group would consist of individuals:
   a Of the same sex, age, and diagnostic category.
   b Of both sexes, different cultural backgrounds, and similar verbal skills.
   c Of the same sex, different ages, and different behavioral patterns.
   d Of both sexes, different diagnostic categories, and the same cultural background.

8 In group therapy, the maximum therapeutic effect tends to occur if the members:
   a Learn to know and trust each other and the leader.
   b Share and participate equally in the interactions.
   c Experience all four phases of group development.
   d All of the above.

9 Every group progresses through developmental phases, each of which is unique and different from the others. The working phase is *best* characterized by:

a Mistrust.

b Competition.

c Apathy.

d Cohesiveness.

10 Which one of the following phases of group development is experienced *most* fully by all groups?

a Preaffiliation.

b Intragroup conflict.

c Working.

d Termination.

11 Ten withdrawn and regressed clients had been assembled for a group experience. Which one of the following groups would be *most* suitable to their needs?

a Psychodrama.

b Socialization.

c Encounter.

d Sensitivity.

12 The lessening of emotional trauma by reenacting the situation is a definition of:

a Catharsis.

b Desensitization.

c Abreaction.

d Ventilation.

13 The method of treatment that helps clients analyze and improve their patterns of interaction by using the child-parent-adult framework is called:

a Insight psychotherapy.

b Transactional analysis.

c Gestalt therapy.

d Psychodrama.

14 Emphasis on the client as a holistic being is *most* specific to which one of the following therapies?

a Transactional analysis.

b Socialization groups.

c Psychodrama.

d Gestalt therapy.

15 A person with substantial ego strength would be a candidate for a group with which one of the following goals?

a Emotional support.

b Remotivation.

c Socialization.

d Emotional insight.

26 *Family theory and intervention*

INTRODUCTION

To define the family in the traditional way as two or more persons related by blood or legal ties is obsolete. Today's family might best be defined as a system composed of human beings of various ages and sexes who are joined together, sometimes by blood or legal ties but often not, for the pursuit of common goals of growth, development, and support of its members.

The view of the family as a system of interrelated parts, one part affecting the others, has major implications for nursing. It suggests that care of sick individuals needs to be expanded to include the other family members who may not demonstrate dysfunctional behaviors but who, nonetheless, are affecting the sick individual as well as being affected by him or her. Intervention would be based on the belief that it is not just one individual who is sick but rather the family system that is experiencing major difficulties functioning. The identified client in the family may be a scapegoat, a victim who helps the other family members maintain a precarious balance. Removing the sick person from the family, even removing the sickness from the individual through treatment measures, may upset the system's homeokinesis and precipitate dysfunctional responses in other members of the family. It seems reasonable, therefore, that all members of the family should be exposed to a therapeutic experience to help them deal more effectively with their complex interrelated problems and stressors.

"Three of the earliest proponents of family therapy were Nathan W. Ackerman at Columbia University, Gerald Caplan at Harvard, and Don Jackson at the University of California. Their earliest work was done in the 1950s. Since that time many theorists have studied the family as a system, and currently there is general agreement that effective promotion of mental health and prevention and treatment of mental illness must take place within a family context. What remains as an unresolved dilemma is how to deliver this type of care within a health delivery system designed to focus on the individual."*

* From Taylor CM: Mereness' essentials of psychiatric nursing, ed 13, St Louis, 1990, The CV Mosby Co, chap 26.

251

The exercises in this chapter are designed to help you review some basic material about the nature of families and their functions and to develop a beginning understanding of the goals of family therapy.

OBJECTIVES

1. To list the functions of the family.
2. To discuss the goals and family dynamics associated with each of the stages of family development.
3. To identify different types of families.
4. To differentiate between effective and ineffective families.
5. To list physical and behavioral manifestations of physical and sexual abuse, physical neglect, and emotional maltreatment commonly observed in abused and neglected children.
6. To list the basic goals of family therapy.

EXERCISES

1 List seven functions of the family.

a _____

b _____

c _____

d _____

e _____

f _____

g _____

2 Using the following grid, identify the onset, list the goals, and describe the family dynamics associated with the seven stages of family development. Phase one of stage one has been filled in to help you get started.

Stages	Onset	Goal	Family dynamics
I	Phase one: Begins when a childless couple makes a commitment to each other.	To adjust to living together as a married pair.	Stressful period. Couple strives to effect a union and learns to assume the roles of husband and wife without losing their individuality.
	Phase two:		
II			
III			
IV			
V			
VI			
VII			

3 Listed below are twenty examples of family groupings. Categorize each one in terms of one of the four family types it represents by placing a check in the box in the appropriate column. The first one has been filled in to help you get started.

	Types of families			
Family groupings	Blended family*	Extended family	Household concept	Nuclear family
1. A man and a woman joined together for the purpose of bearing and raising children.	☐	☐	☐	☑
2. A union of a man and a woman who bring children from previous marriages into the relationship.	☐	☐	☐	☐
3. A man, his children, and the paternal grandmother living together.	☐	☐	☐	☐
4. A man and a woman living together and raising an adopted child.	☐	☐	☐	☐
5. A gay couple, each divorced, living together with children from their straight marriages.	☐	☐	☐	☐
6. A two-generation family consisting of parents and children.	☐	☐	☐	☐
7. A man and two women, living together in an asexual relationship, for emotional support and financial benefit.	☐	☐	☐	☐
8. A widow living with her parents.	☐	☐	☐	☐
9. Several men and women living together in a group home for the purpose of emotional support.	☐	☐	☐	☐
10. Two divorced persons raising children from their previous marriages with children from the current union.	☐	☐	☐	☐
11. Four generations of great-grandparents, grandparents, children and their spouses, and offspring living and working together on a farm.	☐	☐	☐	☐
12. Grandparents raising their grandchildren.	☐	☐	☐	☐
13. Two or more people living together and building a relationship based on mutual respect and interests rather than procreation.	☐	☐	☐	☐
14. Multiple generations related by blood, living together, pooling resources, sharing labor, and giving affection and support to each other.	☐	☐	☐	☐
15. A divorced man raising his son alone.	☐	☐	☐	☐
16. A group of people bonded together in pursuit of a common goal: growth and development of its members.	☐	☐	☐	☐
17. A widow and widower, retired and unmarried to each other, living together with respect and companionship, collecting separate pensions and Social Security benefits.	☐	☐	☐	☐
18. A married couple, their children, and the maternal grandparents living together under one roof.	☐	☐	☐	☐
19. A widow and widower, each with two children from their first marriages, raising them together with two newly adopted children.	☐	☐	☐	☐
20. A couple temporarily raising several foster children, none of whom are related.	☐	☐	☐	☐

*Also known as reconstituted family.

4 Listed on p. 254 are fifteen characteristics of effective and ineffective families. Differentiate between them by placing a check in the box in the appropriate column. The first one has been filled in to help you get started.

Characteristics	Families	
	Effective	Ineffective
1. Promotes cohesive patterns of relating.	☑	☐
2. Adapts to changes within and outside the family without loss of stability.	☐	☐
3. Fosters overt hostility between its members.	☐	☐
4. Manifests learning difficulties and antisocial behaviors in its children.	☐	☐
5. Accepts differences between its members.	☐	☐
6. Works together to deal effectively with problems as they arise.	☐	☐
7. Scapegoats the most powerless family member.	☐	☐
8. Exposes its young people to experiences perpetuating the effective family model.	☐	☐
9. Exhibits chronic patterns of dissension.	☐	☐
10. Maintains stability in the face of changes inside and outside the family group.	☐	☐
11. Manifests tensions in domestic violence.	☐	☐
12. Emphasizes material needs over emotional, physical, and social needs.	☐	☐
13. Strives for power by abusing or neglecting its children.	☐	☐
14. Promotes decision making appropriate to the needs of its members.	☐	☐
15. Provides mutual support and respect for its members.	☐	☐

5 One of the increasingly common symptoms of ineffective families is the abuse or neglect of one of its weaker members. Often this victim is a child. As caretakers who come in contact with children in a variety of health-related as well as non-health-related settings, it is imperative that nurses be alert to both the physical and behavioral indications of child abuse and neglect so that appropriate action can be taken. The following exercise has two parts. First, list in the four columns at least twelve different manifestations of physical abuse, physical neglect, sexual abuse, and emotional maltreatment of children. Second, differentiate between physical and behavioral manifestations by placing a letter "P" or "B" after each one. The first one in each column has been filled in to help you get started.

Physical abuse	Physical neglect	Sexual abuse	Emotional maltreatment
1. Vacant stare (B)	Underweight (P)	Pregnancy (P)	Rocking (B)
2.			
3.			
4.			
5.			
6.			
7.			
8.			
9.			
10.			
11.			
12.			

6 List four basic goals of family therapy:

a _____

b _____

c _____

d _____

DIRECTIONS: Select the *best* response. (Answers appear in the Appendix.)

1 *All but which one* of the following individuals was an early proponent of family therapy?

a Nathan Ackerman.   c Clifford Beers.

b Gerald Caplan.   d Don Jackson.

2 A grouping of several blood-related generations living together under one roof is an example of which one of the following type families?

a Reconstituted.   c Blended.

b Extended.   d Nuclear.

3 The traditional definition of the family is one in which two or more people are:

a Joined in the pursuit of common goals.

b Living together for purposes of procreation.

c Related by blood or legal ties.

d Associated for protection and support.

4 One of the *most* significant aspects of the family's function of regulation of sexual activity and reproduction is the:

a Transmission of cultural heritage.

b Proliferation of sex education.

c Promotion of "safe sex."

d Control of venereal disease.

5 The first stage of family development concludes with the married couple:

a Renewing their marriage vows.

b Testing out their roles of husband and wife.

c Exploring and discovering each other.

d Adjusting to the wife's pregnancy.

6 The "launching" stage of family development refers to which one of the following tasks?

a Children entering school for the first time.

b Children leaving home to start their own family.

c Parents learning the grandparent role.

d Parents facing retirement and postretirement years.

7 The postparental family is faced with which one of the following tasks?

a Preparing the children to leave home.

b Adapting to dissolution of the family.

c Adjusting to the "empty nest syndrome."

d Retiring from full-time employment.

8 The union of two persons and their children from two previous marriages is an example of which one of the following family types?

   a Nuclear.   c Household.

   b Reconstituted.   d Extended.

9 The criterion used by the U.S. Census Bureau to define a family is based on people:

   a Living together under the same roof.

   b United by legal commitment.

   c Related by blood.

   d Having similar interests and goals.

10 Which of the following *best* characterizes an effective family?

   a Placing emotional, physical, and social needs over material possessions.

   b Making and carrying out decisions appropriate to the family's goals.

   c Recognizing, valuing, and accepting the differences among members.

   d All of the above.

11 *Most* ineffective families are characterized by:

   a Child neglect.   c Divorce.

   b Irresolvable stress.   d Violence.

12 Which one of the following is a *physical indicator* of emotional maltreatment in children?

   a Speech disorders.   c Attempted suicide.

   b Unexplained burns.   d Poor hygiene.

13 Child abuse is more common in which one of the following types of families?

   a Single-parent family.   c Extended family.

   b Blended family.   d Nuclear family.

14 According to the systems theory approach to intervention with families:

   a Removal of the deviant member of the family will restore family homeokinesis.

   b Exposure of the sick family member to group interaction will interfere with group equilibrium.

   c Treatment of the deviant member separate from the other members is rarely effective.

   d Support of the sick member will sanction dysfunctional responses in other members.

15 The treatment of choice to use with a married couple in the first stage of family development is:

   a Crisis intervention.   c Group therapy.

   b Conjoint therapy.   d Family therapy.

Section five word games and section exercises

1 Matching: Historical perspective

DIRECTIONS: Listed below are the names of ten persons who have contributed significantly to the fields of psychiatry and psychiatric–mental health nursing. Also listed are their contributions. Match the person with the contribution by placing the number of the contribution in the space provided by the contributor. The first one has been filled in to help you get started. (The solution appears in the Appendix.)

Contributions	Contributors
1. Developed and used psychodrama in the treatment of emotionally disturbed individuals.	___ Ackerman
2. Wrote on the subject of domestic violence.	___ Bales
3. Was a proponent of conjoint family therapy.	___ Berne
4. Developed and used gestalt therapy.	___ Caplan
5. Instituted crisis therapy with military personnel in World War II.	___ Duvall
6. Identified roles assumed by individuals in group situations.	___ Feldman
7. Promoted and used family therapy.	___ Menninger
8. Developed a theory explaining the onset of a crisis in a healthy person.	_1_ Moreno
9. Outlined a series of stages characterizing family development.	___ Perls
10. Developed the theory of transactional analysis.	___ Satir

2 Word search

DIRECTIONS: Listed below are fifty-seven words hidden in the puzzle grid. They may be read up or down, forward or backward, or diagonally, but always in a straight line. Some words may overlap and some letters in the grid may be used more than once. Not all the letters in the grid will be used. Circle each word as you locate it. One word has been circled to help you get started. (The solution appears in the Appendix.)

```
I N T E R V E N T I O N S S E N E V I S E H O C S
N O I T N E V E R P P R O T E C T I O N R N J I E
I I O E S C A P E R E M O T I V A T I O N O S T L
T T R E D R O C E R Z N A N X I E T Y I X I P D F
I C D I S E Q U I L I B R I U M X P A T R S O P L
A E S I F F U E R S N Z D O G E T L O C S N R E I
T F E N V A E P B A A R E J E C T E R N S E I D M
O F M T G O U A P S G U L N O I Y S Z U A T Y O I
R A A I G R R O R U R E O O B L P S U F M A F R T
I P O M U A V C O B O T R C S U P U F S D L U A I
E S T A I E T H E G E L C H O R T I N Y S L V G N
N Y C C D L S I C R R A B R X P L F E D E B C K G
T C E Y A C Y L O O N I G T R I I S E S N E F E D
E H L O N U L D H U I N U B A C H N B L O C K E R
R O G T C N A O C P S E F T T B U D G E S T A L T
E D E X T E N D E D I E R T U X N A L O S S A
B R N O Y P A R E H T O N S W A M S P D D U M B E
M A D U L T C B L E N D E D G H U J E E Y R G G R
E M O T I O N S R E Z I G R E N E M Y R O Z I J H
M A I N T E R A C T I O N W N O I T A N I M R E T
```

ABUSE	ENCOURAGER	NUCLEAR
ADULT	ENERGIZER	ORIENTER
AFFECTION	ESCAPE	PREAFFILIATION
ANXIETY	EXTENDED	PREVENTION
BLENDED	FAMILY	PROTECTION
BLOCKER	FEAR	PSYCHODRAMA
CATALYST	GESTALT	RECORDER
CHILD	GOAL	REJECTER
COHESIVENESS	GROUPS	REMOTIVATION
CONJOINT	GUIDANCE	REORGANIZE
COPING	INITIATOR	ROLE
CRISIS	INTERACTION	RULES
DEFENSES	INTERVENTIONS	SELF-LIMITING
DENIAL	INTIMACY	SUBGROUP
DISEQUILIBRIUM	LEADER	TENSION
DIVORCE	LOSS	TERMINATION
DYAD	MEMBER	THERAPY
DYSFUNCTIONS	NEGLECT	THREAT
EMOTIONS	NORMS	TRAUMA

3 Logic problem

DIRECTIONS: Bette, Lawrence, Dexter, Frank, and Janet are all clients who come to the community mental health center (CMHC) and participate in five different multidisciplinary therapies. Each client comes on a different evening during the week. Using the clues and the grid provided below, match the clients with the appropriate therapy and the evening they attend their sessions.

Clues:

- **a** Bette goes to family therapy three evenings before Frank goes to his session.
- **b** Psychodrama is held on Thursday evening.
- **c** Lawrence participates in conjoint therapy with his wife.
- **d** Janet had attended both psychodrama and gestalt therapy in the past but is now involved in a different therapy.
- **e** Frank's choice of program was partly limited by the fact that he could only come to the CMHC on Tuesday or Thursday evenings.
- **f** Dexter goes to his therapy session on Wednesday evening.
- **g** Gestalt therapy is held the evening after transactional analysis.

(Use an X in the boxes as you rule out a therapy program or evening for each client, an O when you identify a therapy program or evening you think is appropriate for the client. For example, in the grid Dexter has an O filled in for Wednesday (since he attends the program on that evening—Clue f) and Xs for all the four other evenings (since by process of elimination he would not be in programs on any other evening.)

(The solution appears in the Appendix.)

Grid:	Therapies					Evenings of the week				
Clients	FT	P	CT	GT	TA	M	T	W	Th	F
Bette										
Lawrence										
Dexter						X	X	O	X	X
Frank										
Janet										
Mon										
Tues										
Wed										
Thur										
Fri										

Clients (left label for first five rows)
Evenings of the week (left label for last five rows)

259

ANSWERS TO EXERCISES AND TEST ITEMS AND SOLUTIONS TO WORD
GAMES AND SECTION EXERCISES

Answers to exercises

CHAPTER 1

Exercise 1   Prehistoric: 1, 2. Greek-Roman: 3, 4. Middle Ages: 5. Sixteenth and seventeenth centuries: 6, 7. Eighteenth century: 8, 9. Nineteenth century: 10, 11, 12, 13. Twentieth century: 14, 15, 16, 17, 18, 19, 20.

Exercise 2   To serve people residing in catchment area; to assist community improve its level of mental health; to return hospitalized individuals to community living; to help hospitalized individuals maintain family and community ties.

Exercise 3   2: Emphasize group rather than one-to-one intervention methods. 3: Utilize services of individuals already working in the catchment area served by the center. 4: Advocate an interdisciplinary approach to treatment. 5: Strive to promote social change within the community served by the center. 6: Utilize methods of prevention of mental illness.

Exercise 4   Clinical psychologist: 6, 10. Psychiatric social worker: 3, 8. Psychiatrist: 1, 2, 5. Activity therapist: 4, 7, 9.

CHAPTER 2

Exercise 1   Individual admits and discharges him/herself via own signature.

Exercise 2   Emergency commitment: An individual who is clearly dangerous to him/herself or to others is hospitalized for 3 to 5 days for observation. Temporary commitment: The individual is involuntarily hospitalized for a longer period of time, generally up to six months time. Extended or indefinite commitment: An individual is hospitalized against his/her will for an unspecified period of time.

Exercise 3   Marrying; getting a divorce; making telephone calls; keeping personal belongings; making contracts; writing and mailing letters; making purchases; pursuing an education; making a will; getting a job; following religious practices.

Exercise 4   Right to habeas corpus: 1, 7, 8. Right to treatment: 3, 9, 13. Right to informed consent: 2, 6, 14. Right to confidentiality/privacy: 11. Right to independent psychiatric examination: 5. Right to refuse treatment: 10, 15. Right to be free of restraints: 4, 12.

CHAPTER 3

Exercise 1   Discussion.

Exercise 2   Personal examples.

CHAPTER 4

Exercise 1   Self-understanding implies an in-depth knowledge about *why* one believes and feels as one does; self-awareness involves being in touch with one's beliefs and feelings without understanding their roots or sources.

Exercise 2   Personal responses.

Exercise 3a   Personal responses.

Exercise 3b   Discussion, experiences, role playing.

CHAPTER 5

Exercise 1   Holistic being: 4, 8, 13. Strengths and assets: 1, 12, 14, 19, 22. Unique human being: 2, 7, 15, 16. Potential for relating: 3, 11, 17, 25. Behavior communicates: 5, 10. Learn effective adaptations: 9, 18, 20, 21, 23, 24. Quality interactions: 6, 11.

Exercise 2   To develop a more positive concept of self; to develop a more harmonious pattern of interpersonal relationships; to assume a more productive role in society.

CHAPTER 6

Exercise 1   1: Expressing one's thoughts and feelings in writing. 2: Expressing one's thoughts and feelings through the spoken word; 3: Also referred to as body language because one's thoughts and feelings are expressed through facial expression, quality and tone of voice, posture, and gestures. 4: The role expectation individuals have of one another in the context in which verbal and nonverbal communication occurs.

Exercise 2   Initiating a conversation: 1, 2, 3, 8, 9, 11. Getting information: 2, 9. Establishing rapport: 3, 15. Encouraging expression of feelings and thoughts: 5, 6, 12. Arriving at a decision: 5, 13. Providing reassurance: 6, 12. Stimulating interest: 4, 10. Concluding a conversation: 7, 14.

Exercise 3   Effective: 2, 3, 6, 7, 10. Ineffective: 1, 4, 5, 8, 9.

Exercise 4   Clarifying: 4, 7. Encouraging: 8, 10. Exploring: 22. Focusing: 6, 22. Giving information: 1, 2, 5, 14, 20, 21. Introducing neutral topic: 18. Making observations: 3, 6. Reflecting: 3, 4, 11, 13. Seeking information: 12. Suggesting: 17. Understanding: 9, 13, 15, 16, 19.

Exercise 5   Therapeutic: 1: Sitting during conversation, reaching out, touching, nodding head; 2: Presenting a quiet, calm, unhurried, mild, soft-spoken manner: 3: Smiling, natural eye contact. Nontherapeutic: 1: Standing during conversation, restlessness, shifting on feet, touching, pointing, shaking finger; 2: Using a loud, challenging, sharp tone and short, abrupt responses: 3: Avoiding eye contact, looking around in distracted manner during conversation, frowning, grimacing, smiling. (It should be noted that even therapeutic approaches may have nontherapeutic effects. For example, a suspicious person may be threatened by touching and reaching out, or a smile may be distorted and misinterpreted. Cultural differences may also be a factor in how nonverbal approaches are perceived. For example, Chinese clients find the nurses' "hovering" comforting and reassuring, while other cultural groups might misinterpret such attention as an indication that they are very sick and might find it anxiety producing.)

Exercise 1	Emergency interventions: 4, 6, 8, 12. Brief associations: 2, 5, 9, 14. Long-term relationships: 1, 3, 7, 10, 11, 13, 15.
Exercise 2	Orientation: 1: Getting acquainted period; nurse and client are strangers to each other. 2: To develop trust; to establish the nurse as significant to the client. 3: Usually initiated by nurse who seeks out client, introduces self, and offers to work with the client; accepts testing behaviors; responds with consistency. Maintenance: 1: Working phase characterized by nurse and client actively working together on client's problems. 2: To identify and resolve the client's problems. 3: Nurse focuses on client's problems; sets limits on behaviors as necessary; encourages expression of fears, concerns, hopes, problems. Termination: 1: Concluding phase in which nurse and client prepare for end of the relationship. 2: To help client review learnings that came out of the relationship; to transfer learnings to interactions with others. 3: Nurse deals with client's response to termination: denial, regression, dependency, rebellion; encourages client to express anger, depression, loss associated with ending; nurse deals with own feelings associated with termination.
Exercise 3a	Approaches client; introduces self by name; asks client's name and checks out how she would like to be addressed; suggests working together; identifies purpose of the meetings; suggests time and place to meet; uses communication skills, including introducing a neutral topic until client's needs and problems are identified; responds consistently, adhering to schedule of meetings; accepts testing behaviors; sets limits on behaviors as necessary.
Exercise 3b	Meeting hygiene needs; expressing feelings appropriately; relating; weight control; controlling impulses such as eating, masturbation, aggression.
Exercise 3c	Accepting: 1, 3, 4, 6, 7, 10, 12, 13, 14, 15. Nonaccepting: 2, 5, 8, 9, 11.
Exercise 3d	Consistent/therapeutic: 1, 2, 5, 6, 7, 9, 10, 11, 12, 15. Inconsistent/nontherapeutic: 3, 4, 8, 13, 14.
Exercise 4	Social: 2, 5, 7, 9, 10. Therapeutic: 1, 3, 4, 6, 8.
Exercise 5	2: Respond in an honest, sincere, caring, friendly manner; communicate expectation that client can change. 3: Encourage common social and work activities in groups—conversation, singing, ward chores, arts and crafts, eating, games. 4: Demonstrate, orient, and instruct client in activities of daily living; set limits as necessary. 5: Temporarily assume parenting activities for clients who are too ill to take responsibility—bathing, dressing, toileting, feeding, and limit setting. 6: Collaborate with others on the health team in developing and implementing a treatment plan; initiate and promote a therapeutic nurse-client relationship. 7: Provide helpful, realistic reassurance—respond with consistency, sit with client, and listen in an interested and empathic way.
Exercise 6	Keep tray of medications inaccessible to ambulatory clients; administer medications to one client at a time; observe for side effects, adverse effects, and changes in behavior; use opportunity to interact with client; respond to client's questions about medications; report and record nursing interventions effective in getting resistant client to take medications; teach clients about medications preparatory to discharge if they are to be maintained on drugs.

CHAPTER 8

Exercise 1 Physical Environment: Therapeutic: 2, 5, 6, 11. Nontherapeutic: 1, 8, 10, 13, 17, 19. Socioemotional climate: Therapeutic: 3, 9, 12, 15, 18. Nontherapeutic: 4, 7, 14, 16, 20.

Exercise 2 Personal responses.

Exercise 3 Play Ping-Pong with clients; move chairs into conversational circle around the low table and encourage interaction; sit with three clients at the table for four and play a table game from the bookcase; facilitate a sing-along around the piano; encourage orientation by focusing on the clock, calendar; post schedules of activities, birthdays, news items, client's art work on the bulletin board; place plants on the window sills and bookcase and encourage clients to care for them; refer to books and magazines when interacting; form discussion circle near the TV and encourage discussion of a program that has just been viewed.

Exercise 4 Provide favorable climate in which client can gain self-awareness; try new interpersonal skills; focus more on others and less on self; develop self-esteem; appraise potentially helpful and destructive aspects of behavior; practice decision making; participate in group activities and group decisions.

CHAPTER 9

Exercise 1 Activity: 1, 2, 10. Cognition: 9, 15. Ecological: 3. Emotional: 4. Interpersonal: 5, 6, 14. Perception: 11, 12. Physiological: 8, 13. Valuation: 7.

Exercise 2a Direct observation, client interview, medic alert records, previous hospital records, neighbors, police.

Exercise 2b Seeing: 1, 3, 4, 7, 8. Hearing: 2, 6, 9. Smelling: 5, 10. Touching: 4, 8.

Exercise 2c ANA Diagnostic Framework: 1.3.4 Altered Self Care R/T confusion, 2.5.2.4 Memory Deficit R/T confusion, 5.4.2 Altered Family Processes R/T confusion, 5.7.2 Altered Social Interaction R/T confusion, 7.9.2.2 Altered Skin Integrity R/T confusion. NANDA Diagnostic Framework: 1.6.2.1.2.1 Impaired Skin Integrity R/T confusion, 3.1.2 Social Isolation R/T confusion, 3.2.2 Altered Family Processes R/T confusion, 6.5.2 Bathing/Hygiene/Self Care Deficit R/T confusion, 6.5.3 Dressing/Grooming Self Care Deficit R/T confusion, 6.5.4 Toileting Self Care Deficit R/T confusion.

Exercise 2d Technical role: 4, 7. CTE: 8. Socializing agent: 1, 10. Teacher: 3. Parent surrogate: 3, 9. Nurse therapist: 2, 5. Counselor: 2, 5, 6.

Exercise 2e To orient the client to the identity of the nurse and the purpose of the interview; to ascertain client's perception of his or her problems; to determine duration of the problem; to obtain factual information about the client's ADL, previous health history, etc.

Exercise 2f 2: "What are you frowning about?" 3: "Where is the pain?" "How long does the pain last?" 4: "What do you usually eat for breakfast . . .?" 5: "What is your daughter's name?" "Where does your daughter live?" "When did you see her last?" 6: "How many hours do you sleep at night?" "Do you take pills to help you sleep?" 7: "What has happened to upset you?" 8: "How did you get those bruises on your arms?" 9: "Who are your neighbors?" 10: "How do you feel about returning to the boardinghouse?"

CHAPTER 10

Exercise 1	Family: 2, 6, 11. Social: 3, 10, 14. Community: 4, 8, 9, 15. Physiological: 1, 5, 13. Psychological: 7, 12.
Exercise 2	Open: 1, 2, 5, 8, 9, 11, 12, 13, 14, 15. Closed: 3, 4, 6, 7, 10.
Exercise 3	Developmental: 2, 4, 5, 9, 10, 11, 13. Situational: 1, 3, 6, 7, 8, 12, 14, 15.
Exercise 4	Personal examples.

CHAPTER 11

Exercise 1	Self-acceptance; realistic perception of reality; environmental mastery; independent thinking and behaving (problem solving, autonomy, self-determination); synthesizing all psychological functions and personal attributes leading to unified, integrated outlook on life and goal-directed behavior.
Exercise 2a	1: Directs rational, thoughtful behavior; concerned with thoughts, feelings, and sensations; aware of here and now. 2: Storage area for memories that can be recalled at will; keeps disturbing material out of consciousness. 3: Largest storage area for memories; content cannot be recalled at will.
Exercise 2b	Id: 1, 5, 8, 10, 13, 15. Ego: 2, 3, 6, 11. Superego: 4, 7, 9, 12, 14.
Exercise 2c	1: Other pleasurable activities: crying, chewing, swallowing. 2: Anus, urethra: Evacuation of bladder and bowels. 3: Immature genitalia: Manipulation of genitalia (masturbation). 4: None: Stable, dormant stage. Child finds pleasure associating with other children, in acquiring skills and knowledge. 4: Mature genitalia: Genital-to-genital activity with partner of opposite sex.
Exercise 3	1-h, 2-p, 3-n, 4-j, 5-o, 6-d, 7-l, 8-g, 9-k, 10-a, 11-e, 12-c, 13-m, 14-f, 15-b, 16-i.
Exercise 4a	2: Strives for and learns to use power: Child feels beginning sense of power related to attempts to control self and others. 3: Acquires and uses universal language: Child gives up personal language and uses universal language as a tool to promote relationships; able to consensually validate perceptions and feelings with others. 4: Learns to compete and compromise: Child turns away from adults and turns to peers of same sex. Tests out tools of competition and compromise. Peers reinforce or alter child's self-concept. 5: Forms close relationship with chum: Continues group affiliations while developing an intimate relationship with one special friend of the same sex. Significant adults outside the family impact on child's concept of self. 6: Experiences lust: In response to sexual urges, adolescent turns to peers of the opposite sex while continuing to be influenced by peer group of the same sex. 7: Integration of intimacy and lust: Adolescent integrates intimacy and lust into mature adult relationship with person of the opposite sex.
Exercise 4b	Good-me: 1, 4, 8, 9, 13, 15. Bad-me: 2, 3, 6, 7, 11. Not-me: 5, 10, 12, 14.
Exercise 4c	Good-me: 2, 8, 9, 10, 13. Bad-me: 1, 3, 5, 7, 11, 14. Not-me: 4, 6, 12, 15.
Exercise 5	Sensorimotor: 2, 5, 6. P/P: 1, 9. P/I: 4. Concrete: 8, 10. Formal: 3, 7.

CHAPTER 12

Exercise 1	Intrapsychic: 2, 4, 6, 8. Interpersonal: 1, 3, 5, 7, 9, 10.
Exercise 2a	Personal examples.
Exercise 2b	Personal examples.

Exercise 3	2: Isolation. 3: Pleading sick. 4: Somnolent detachment. 5: Suppression. 6: Drinking. 7: Apathy. 8: Undoing. 9: Identification. 10: Problem solving. 11: Pacing. 12: Symbolization/condensation. 13: Reaction formation. 14: Projection. 15: Talking. 16: Denial. 17: Eating. 18: Preoccupation. 19: Regression. 20: Sublimation. 21: Repression. 22: Compensation. 23: Selective inattention. 24: Smoking. 25: Rationalization.

CHAPTER 13

Exercise 1	a: French neurologist who inspired others to conduct formal research into the cause and nature of nervous and mental disorders. b: Psychiatrist whose psychosexual theory of personality development was based on a biological model and revolutionized the understanding of human behavior. c: One of the pioneers in using the scientific method to study genetics as a determinant of mental illness, is best known for his twin studies. d: Two of the first researchers to explore the effect of antipsychotic drugs on the brain.
Exercise 2	Family: 2, 4, 7, 9. Twin: 1, 4, 8. Adoption: 3, 5, 10. Genetic linkage: 6.
Exercise 3	a: The dopamine hypothesis suggests that schizophrenia results from an overactivity of dopamine, a neurotransmitter, in the mesolimbic and mesocortical tracts of the brain. These two tracts are associated with intellectual and emotional functioning, and some symptoms in schizophrenia are thought to involve these two tracts. Antipsychotic medications are thought to block dopamine activity in the brain and have a therapeutic effect on controlling these symptoms. b: The catecholamine hypothesis suggests that catecholamines, another group of neurotransmitters, contribute to the onset of manic-depressive behaviors. It is further thought that a deficiency of catecholamine, particularly norepinephrine, is a factor in the onset of depression, whereas the overactivity in mania may be related to an excess of catecholamine in the brain.
Exercise 4	CT: 1, 2, 3, 5, 6, 7, 8, 10, 11. PET: 1, 4, 7, 9, 12. MRI: 1, 5, 6, 7, 8.

CHAPTER 14

Exercise 1	1: Culture. 2: Cultural norms. 3: Deviance. 4: Cultural stereotyping. 5: Cultural sensitivity. 6: Ethnic group. 7: Social drift. 8: Gender.
Exercise 2	When did you come to this country? With what ethnic or racial group do you identify? Do you live in a neighborhood that supports your cultural orientation? If so, how? Who constitutes your immediate family? What cultural rituals and customs do you follow? What cultural restrictions do you observe? What cultural customs of this country have you adopted? Rejected? What languages do you speak? Read? Write? What are your food preferences? Have you ever been hospitalized before? In this country? If so, did you find anything about being hospitalized troubling? How do you feel about being hospitalized? How do you feel about being cared for by strangers? How do you feel about being touched by strangers? Persons of same sex? Persons of opposite sex?
Exercise 3	1: Utilize family therapy as a treatment modality. 2: Check with family members to learn if client is having pain, experiencing problems, etc., since client may hesitate to share this information with the nurse. 3: Listen to client's beliefs and do not automatically assume that thoughts different from the nurse's are delusional or indicative of mental illness. 4: Show patience and understanding and work at developing a trusting relationship with clients to facilitate communication. 5: Reach out and offer care. 6: Follow up and offer support and encouragement for pursuing treatment goals; utilize short-term crisis-oriented therapy.

CHAPTER 15

Exercise 1	Disorganized: 1, 7, 10, 11, 14. Catatonic: 1, 2, 3, 5, 13, 14, 15. Paranoid: 4, 8, 9, 12, 14. Chronic Undifferentiated: may exhibit any and all behaviors except #6, Residual: 6, 14.
Exercise 2a	Penny learned early in life that relating is anxiety provoking. She experienced a series of rejections beginning in infancy. Her father abandoned both her and her mother. The mother gave up Penny to foster homes. One can speculate that Penny experienced further rejection, inconsistency, double-bind communication, indifference, predominantly negative reflected appraisals, and high anxiety in these homes. Peers (chums) ridiculed her. To defend herself from further anxiety-producing relationships, Penny withdrew into solitary activities. These early experiences laid the foundation for her subsequent difficulties relating, such as in work situations.
Exercise 2b	1: (2) Suspicious, believes she is being poisoned, does not share; (6) sits alone facing door, responds with anger when approached; (12) continues to be suspicious and accuses staff of poisoning her. 2: (4) Wears old clothes and feels different from others; (7) takes no responsibility for her own hygiene, disheveled; (8) negativistic, refuses to follow suggestions, and does the opposite of what is expected. 3: (5) Feels guilty and punishes herself for losing job and not helping mother; (7) unable to make decisions; (9) chants "Dear God, forgive her . . . ". 4: (11) Never completes anything she starts, has difficulty concentrating on tasks, expresses feelings of inadequacy. 5: (9) Refers to herself in the third person; (10) fails to respond to her name, appears not to know her own name, refers to herself as "Nobody". 6: (3) No friends, pursues solitary activities.
Exercise 2c	2: associative looseness, 3: persecutory delusions, 4: auditory hallucinations, 5: regression, 6: flat affect, 7: autism, 8: somatic delusions, 9: psychomotor retardation, 10: negativism, 11: inappropriate affect/behavior, 12: mutism, 13: ambivalence, 14: delusions of grandeur, 15: psychomotor activity.
Exercise 2d	Nursing actions: 1: Seek out client and initiate a positive, corrective, nurse-client relationship; communicate respect by calling her by her correct name; introduce her to others, using her name; point out reality when she calls herself "Nobody". 2: Help client with her hygiene and appearance; provide client with privacy when carrying out hygiene; give positive feedback when client appears tidy and takes initiative in meeting her own needs; encourage her to look in the mirror and begin self-appraisal; gradually encourage her to take responsibility for her own care, to make simple decisions about what to wear. 3: Communicate honesty and sincerity to client; respond with consistency; initially encourage solitary or one-to-one activities with the nurse rather than group activities with other clients. 4: Listen and, when possible, point out when client's perceptions are false without arguing with her. Provide well-balanced diet including, as much as possible, the client's preferred foods; allow client to serve up her own foods; offer self-contained foods such as hard-boiled eggs in the shell, intact fruit, unopened individual containers of milk and juice, etc.; encourage her to eat in the dining room with other clients. Outcome criteria: Within 4 weeks the client will: 1: Respond consistently to her correct name and call herself "Nobody" with less frequency. 2: Take increasing responsibility for her own hygiene; make simple decisions; respond with relative comfort to positive feedback; take interest and initiative in self-appraisal. 3: Seek out the nurse on her own initiative; show interest and receptivity to group interactions and activities. 4: Begin to give up her beliefs

that the food is contaminated; sit in the dining room and eat her meals with other clients; permit her food to be served from the ward community supply; gain several pounds.

Exercise 3a
1: 1.3.4 Altered Self Care R/T regression. 2: 2.1.2 Altered Decision Making R/T ambivalence; 2.2.2 Altered Judgment R/T weak ego; 2.6.2 Altered Thought Processes R/T delusions. 3: 3.1.2 Altered Community Maintenance R/T narcissism; 3.3.2 Altered Home Maintenance R/T psychomotor retardation. 4: 4.1.4 Flat Affect R/T ambivalence. 5: 5.2.2 Altered Communication Processes R/T autistic thinking; 5.7.2 Altered Social Interaction R/T fear of rejection. 6: 6.4.2 Altered Sensory Perception R/T auditory hallucinations. 7: 7.1.2 Altered Circulation R/T psychomotor retardation; 7.2.2 Altered Elimination Processes R/T psychomotor retardation; 7.7.2 Altered Nutrition Processes R/T feelings of suspiciousness. 8: 8.1.2 Altered Meaningfulness R/T feelings of worthlessness.

Exercise 3b
1: 1.1.2.1 Altered Nutrition: More than body requirements R/T decreased metabolism; 1.1.2.2 Altered Nutrition: Less than body requirements R/T hyperactivity; 1.3.1.1 Constipation R/T improper diet; 1.6.1 Potential for Injury R/T withdrawal from reality. 2: 2.1.1.1 Impaired Verbal Communication R/T autistic thinking. 3: 3.1.1 Impaired Social Interaction R/T fear of rejection; 3.1.2 Social Isolation R/T mistrust. 4: 4.1.1 Spiritual Distress R/T feelings of hopelessness. 5: 5.2.1.1 Noncompliance (not taking prescribed medications) R/T feelings of suspiciousness. 6: 6.1.1.1 Impaired Physical Mobility R/T psychomotor retardation; 6.2.1 Sleep Pattern Disturbance R/T hyperactivity; 6.5.3 Dressing/Grooming Self-Care Deficit R/T low self-esteem. 7: 7.1.1 Body Image Disturbance R/T weak ego boundaries; 7.1.2 Self Esteem Disturbance R/T feelings of worthlessness; 7.2 Sensory/Perceptual Alterations R/T delusions. 8: 8.3 Altered Thought Processes R/T delusions. 9: 9.2.2 Potential for Violence: Self-directed R/T auditory hallucinations; 9.2.2 Potential for Violence: Directed at Others R/T auditory hallucinations; 9.3.1 Anxiety R/T empathized anxiety communicated from another person.

Exercise 4
Classification: Antipsychotic, phenothiazine derivative. Other drugs: chlorpromazine (Thorazine), piperacetazine (Quide), mesoridazine (Serentil), fluphenazine (Prolixin), perphenazine (Trilafon), trifluoperazine (Stelazine). Action: Reduce psychotic symptoms; control excited, overactive individuals; normalize withdrawn, inactive individuals; reduce hallucinations and delusions. Range of dosage/Route: 200 to 800 mg/oral. Contraindications/Precautions: In clients in severe CNS depression, comatose states, or psychotic depression; in clients with severe hypotensive or hypertensive heart disease; use cautiously with persons requiring complete mental acuity. Drug idiosyncrasies: Pigmentary retinopathy can occur in persons taking larger than recommended doses; women have greater tendency to orthostatic hypotension than men. Side and adverse effects and nursing implications for each: Dry mouth/offer fluids, gum, candy; constipation/offer fluids, balanced diet, roughage, laxatives; orthostatic hypotension/ambulate gradually; endocrine changes/diet to regulate weight, reassure client; extrapyramidal changes/dose adjustment, use of antiparkinsonism drug as ordered; photosensitivity/protect from rays of the sun; skin reactions, tardive dyskinesia/withhold drug only after reporting to doctor and there has been medical evaluation; jaundice/report to physician, withhold then discontinue drug; agranulocytosis, leukopenia/check white blood count at regularly scheduled intervals, report symptoms of sore throat and colds, withhold then discontinue drug; ocular changes/maintain client on recommended daily dosage, schedule routine eye

examinations, report signs of eye problems, withhold then discontinue drug; convulsions/use anticonvulsants as ordered with persons having history of seizures. Miscellaneous nursing implications: Keep medications inaccessible to psychotic clients, administer drugs to one client at a time, observe, report, and record any side and adverse effects as well as effect of drug on behavior. Source: Taylor, PDR.

Exercise 5   2-i, 3-c, 4-a, 5-b, 6-i, 7-d, 8-f, 9-e, 10-j, 11-d, 12-g, 13-i, 14-h, 15-d.

CHAPTER 16

Exercise 1   Self-esteem: All. Love object: 7, 8, 13, 14. Independence: 1, 2, 4, 6. Freedom: 1, 2, 13. Physical integrity: 1, 3, 4, 5, 14. Youth: 1, 3, 10. Autonomy: 1, 2, 4, 6, 9. Material possessions: 6, 12, 15.

Exercise 2   Grief or bereavement: Normal, universal, reaction to real loss of tangible or intangible, highly valued object; adaptive process; self-limiting; generally not incapacitating except in early, acute stage; phases include shock and disbelief, awareness, restitution. Depression: Disturbance in mood in response to actual, anticipated, or imagined loss; pathological elaboration of grief; goes beyond grief in duration, intensity; current loss is often symbolic of other past losses; incapacitating; not self-limiting; professional help often required.

Exercise 3   Mania: 2, 3, 5, 8, 9, 12, 13, 15. Depression: 1, 4, 5, 6, 7, 8, 10, 11, 14.

Exercise 4a   a: 9, 12, 14. b: 7, 16, 17, 20, 21. c: 12, 16, 17, 20, 21, 27. d: 2, 5, 12. e: 23, 25, 26, 29. f: 30. g: 1, 4. h: 6, 13. i: 3, 8. j: 4, 5, 10, 11, 13, 15, 18, 19, 22, 24, 28.

Exercise 4b   Depression occurs as a response to a real or imagined loss. With the loss of a trusted nurse the client experiences a loss symbolic of earlier losses (mother) and loss of self-esteem. If the feelings are not worked through, the depression can increase in intensity and duration and may affect subsequent relationships. The client with a history of suicide is also a suicidal risk with this new loss.

Exercise 4c   Nursing actions: 1: Focus on the client; use a variety of therapeutic communication skills to facilitate the client's expressing feelings; listen to expressions of anger without becoming defensive; sit in silence with client when she does not feel like talking. 2: Use therapeutic communication skills to help the client reflect back on the relationship and its positive aspects; refocus on topics not fully explored. 3: Encourage client to identify other persons on the unit with whom she feels comfortable; introduce her to others, as necessary; join group activities; respond consistently and firmly that the relationship is over if and when the client tries to get the nurse to visit, write, etc. Outcome criteria: Within 3 weeks the client will: 1: express a range of emotions regarding the separation, including anger and eventually warm regard for the nurse. 2: review the stages of the nurse-client relationship and reflect on the changes and learnings that have occurred during the association. 3: identify at least one other person on the unit with whom she feels comfortable, will spend less and less time with the departing nurse, and will join group activities with other clients.

Exercise 5   Objective: 2: To protect the client from self-destructive tendencies. 3: To assist client with all aspects of daily living. 4: To increase client's daily food intake. 5: To help client develop a more realistic concept of self. 6: To facilitate client's communication with nurse and others. Nursing actions: 2: Assign a nurse to stay with client at all times; administer antidepressant medications as prescribed; observe, listen, report, and record all cues of continued suicidal ideation; encourage participation in supervised and safe OT/RT activities. 3: Establish a simple daily routine for bathing, grooming, eating, physical activity; give encouragement and reassurance to help client follow schedule; use patience; allow enough time for the activity and do not rush client; provide appropriate rest periods but discourage naps during the day. 4: Identify foods that client prefers, considering ethnic influences; serve small amounts of food at meal times; offer nutritional supplements during day and at bedtime; record amount of food consumed; weigh client weekly. 5: Seek out, spend time with client; call client by name; show genuine interest in client; encourage client to talk about him/herself; help client with hygiene as necessary; give client praise for efforts to help self; provide client with activities he/she can succeed in. 6: Seek out client; sit in silence if client does not wish to talk; reflect client's statements to encourage conversation; focus on neutral topics initially when problem areas have not been identified; encourage participation in small group interactions.

Exercise 6

Objective: 2: To help client control aggressive behaviors. 3: To help client assume greater responsibility for self-care. 4: To promote adequate nutrition. 5: To facilitate appropriate communication patterns. 6: To protect client from injury. Nursing actions: 2: Prevent episodes of aggressiveness by identifying and avoiding situations that precipitate outbursts and by being alert to signs of impending outbursts and intervening early; reduce environmental stimuli by assigning client to a single room that is devoid of drapes, pictures, by avoiding client's participation in competitive games and activities, by providing client with quiet activities such as writing; speak calmly, firmly in simple, short sentences; avoid arguing with client; set limits on aggressive behaviors. 3: Give direct assistance with dressing, hygiene, etc., as necessary; use quiet persuasion to encourage client to participate in self-care activities; provide needed equipment for client to carry out self-care; supervise activities, especially in the bathroom; provide adequate time for self-care activity and do not hurry client. 4: Serve high-caloric meals and between-meal nourishment; feed client in his or her room if dining room is too stimulating or distracting; remain with client and keep client focused on eating; use unbreakable food-serving equipment; provide client with "finger foods", foods that can be held in the hand and eaten while walking about; weigh client weekly and report/record the weight. 5: Talk to client in a firm, low-pitched voice; listen to client's pointed, hostile remarks without becoming defensive; avoid laughing at client's jokes. 6: Administer lithium as prescribed; keep client under close supervision, especially when client is smoking, bathing, eating, participating in arts and crafts activities; check that client is warmly dressed during cold weather.

Exercise 7a

Classification: Antidepressant, tricyclic. Other drugs: imipramine (Tofranil), amitriptyline (Elavil), nortriptyline (Aventyl, Pamelor), doxepin (Sinequan, Adapin). Action: Relief of depression. Range of dosage/Route: 75 to 200 mg/oral. Contraindications/Precautions: In clients with history of cardiovascular disease, urinary retention, glaucoma, thyroid disease, seizures. Drug idiosyncrasies: Effective more quickly than other tricyclics; drug may be stopped and another in the tricyclic family started with no delay; if an MAO inhibitor is to be started, there should be a delay of at least 2 weeks to allow for complete metabolism of the drug and to avoid the development of hypertensive crisis; abrupt cessation of drug after prolonged use may produce nausea, headache, malaise. Side and adverse effects and nursing implications for each: Dry mouth, postural hypotension, perspiration, visual symptoms, tremor, convulsions, twitching, or ataxia/report to the physician; can usually be controlled by reduction in dosage; exacerbation of psychosis, cardiac arrhythmias/report and then discontinue drug. Miscellaneous nursing implications: Client may require several weeks on drug before effect on depression is noted; observe client closely for suicidal ideation and acts during this period. Observe, report, and record any side or adverse effects. Source: Taylor, PDR.

Exercise 7b   Classification: Antidepressant, monoamine oxidase inhibitor (MAO). Other drugs: isocarboxazid (Marplan), phenelzine sulfate (Nardil). Action: Reduces depression. Range of dosage/Route: 20 to 30 mg/oral. Contraindications/Precautions: In clients with cardiovascular disorders, history of liver disease/use under close supervision (generally in hospital) when tricyclics have been ineffective. Drug idiosyncrasies: Potentiates effects of many other substances, including alcohol and barbiturates. Avoid use with other MAOs or tricyclics, drugs containing epinephrine or ephedrine, and foods containing tyramine or excessive caffeine. Side and adverse effects and nursing implications for each: Dry mouth, postural hypotension, perspiration, visual symptoms, tremor, convulsions, twitching, or ataxia/report to the physician; can usually be controlled by reduction in dosage; hypertensive crisis/can be prevented by avoiding specific substances including over-the-counter cold remedies and antihistamines, aged cheese, whiskey, beer, Chianti wine, cream, chocolate, coffee, soy sauce, chicken livers, raisins, yeast products. Miscellaneous nursing implications: Observe client for suicidal ideation and acts during time it takes for drug to be effective, check that client swallows pills and does not save them for suicide attempt. Observe, report, and record any side or adverse effects. Source: Taylor, PDR.

Exercise 7c   Classification: Antimanic. Other drugs: None. Action: Normalizes manic behaviors within 1 to 3 weeks; target symptoms include pressure of speech, hyperactivity, flight of ideas, grandiosity, poor judgment, aggressiveness. Range of dosage/Route: 900 to 1200 mg/oral; dosage is individualized, according to serum levels and clinical response. Contraindications/Precautions: In clients with significant renal or cardiovascular disease, in clients who are severely debilitated, dehydrated, or experiencing sodium depletion, in clients taking diuretics/drug may be contraindicated or used cautiously. Drug idiosyncrasies: Lithium toxicity is closely related to serum lithium levels; the ability to tolerate lithium is greater during acute mania and decreases as manic symptoms decrease. Side and adverse effects and nursing implications for each: Fine hand tremor, polyuria, mild thirst, transient mild nausea are sometimes seen in early treatment/often subside without intervention; if persistent, dosage may need to be adjusted; diarrhea, vomiting, drowsiness, muscular weakness, lack of coordination, giddiness, ataxia, blurred vision, tinnitus, abdominal cramps, and large output of dilute urine/require dosage adjustment; failure to do so may result in renal tubule damage, cardiac toxicity, thyroid imbalance. Miscellaneous nursing implications: Serum levels should be determined twice a week initially, then may be reduced; desirable range is 1.0 to 1.5 mEq/l; toxicity can often be prevented if serum lithium level is kept below 1.5; to counteract the lag period, antipsychotic agents are sometimes used; however, the combined use of haloperidol with lithium may produce encephalopathic syndrome; clients should be maintained on normal diet, including salt, and a fluid intake of 2500 to 3000 ml; outpatients should be instructed about symptoms of toxicity and the need to discontinue drug and notify physician if they occur. Observe, report, and record any side or adverse effects. Source: Taylor, PDR.

CHAPTER 17

Exercise 1	Oral: 2, 5, 6, 7, 11, 13. Anal: 1, 4, 8, 10. Phallic: 3, 9, 12, 14, 15.
Exercise 2a	Id: 1, 2, 6, 9, 10. Ego: 5, 7, 8, 14, 15, 17, 18, 19. SE: 3, 4, 11, 12, 13, 16, 20.

Exercise 2b An individual is born with the id, the source of instinctual drives. It strives to achieve pleasure and to avoid or relieve pain. There is no conflict with gratifying these drives until the ego develops. The ego begins to develop as the individual comes into contact with the environment and reality. It strives to effect a compromise among the demands of the id, reality factors, and, eventually, the ideals of the superego. The superego, the last part of the personality to develop, integrates the taboos, prohibitions, ideals, and standards of parents and other adults in the maturing individual's life. If the superego is too rigid and punitive and the ego is ineffective in setting realistic limits and compromises on instinctual drives, the individual may experience conflict and feelings of anxiety and guilt when primitive, instinctual drives emerge.

Exercise 3 Displacement: 1, 3, 4, 7, 8, 9, 11. Symbolism: 1, 2, 3, 4, 5, 7, 8, 9, 10, 11. Conversion: 2, 5, 10. Preoccupation: 1, 3, 4, 7, 8, 9, 11. Undoing: 1, 4, 8, 11. Repression: all. Dissociation: 6, 12.

Exercise 4 b: Experience obsessive thoughts/preoccupations. c: Fail to maintain home environment or are preoccupied with cleanliness and excessive carrying out of cleanliness rituals. d: Experience feelings of anxiety, guilt, impending doom. e: Alienate themselves from others who fail to understand that their behaviors are a reflection of illness and who grow impatient with their fears, rituals, and physical symptoms. f: Critical of self and their inability to control their obsessive thoughts, compulsive acts. g: Experience physical symptoms such as loss of appetite, sleeplessness, palpitations, shortness of breath, fatigue. h: Experience feelings of helplessness, hopelessness, and powerlessness and may use drugs, alcohol, suicide (all methods outside their value system) to achieve relief.

Exercise 5b Nursing diagnoses: Altered Motor Behavior R/T anxiety stemming from unconscious conflicts (ANA: 1.1.2) or Anxiety R/T unconscious conflicts (NANDA: 9.3.2). Nursing objective: To help decrease client's anxiety. Nursing actions: Administer anxiolytic medications as ordered by the physician, encourage and support client's use of physical exercise/activities as a release of physical tension, listen to client's verbalizations of concerns, tell client about availability of various psychotherapies as tools to gain insight into unconscious conflicts and/or experience support.

Exercise 5c Nursing diagnoses: Altered Recreation Patterns R/T fear of going outdoors (ANA: 1.2.2) or Diversional Activity Deficit R/T fear of going outdoors (NANDA: 6.3.1.1). Nursing objective: To help decrease client's anxiety. Nursing actions: Administer anxiolytic meds as ordered by the physician, accept client's need to restrict activities at this time, encourage client to explore alternate recreational activities to be carried out at home, listen to client's verbalizations of concerns, tell client about availability of various psychotherapies as tools to gain insight into unconscious conflicts and/or experience support.

Exercise 5d Nursing diagnoses: Altered Self Concept R/T feelings of powerlessness (ANA: 6.3.2) or Self Esteem Disturbance R/T feelings of powerlessness (NANDA: 7.1.2) or Powerlessness R/T high levels of anxiety (NANDA: 7.3.2). Nursing objective: To help client develop a more realistic concept of self, to help decrease client's anxiety. Nursing actions: Administer anxiolytic medications as ordered by the physician, listen and accept client's expressions of feelings, call client by name, provide client with activities she can succeed in, encourage client to make reasonable decisions, give mild praise and recognition for client's efforts to help herself, support client's decision to participate in therapy.

Exercise 5e
Nursing diagnoses: Altered Role Performance R/T anxiety stemming from unconscious conflicts (ANA: 5.5.2, NANDA: 3.2.1). Nursing objective: To help decrease client's anxiety. Nursing actions: Administer anxiolytic medications as ordered by the physician, accept client's need to conduct rituals to control anxiety, allow client to carry out ritual without interruption as long as ritual is not life-threatening, provide time needed for client to carry out ritual, listen to client's expressions of concerns, tell client about the availability of various psychotherapies as tools to gain insight into unconscious conflicts and/or experience support.

Exercise 5f
Nursing diagnoses: Fear R/T preoccupation with physical symptoms stemming from severe anxiety (ANA: 4.1.2.5, ANA: 9.3.2). Nursing objective: To help decrease client's anxiety. Nursing actions: Administer anxiolytic medications as ordered by the physician, focus on client, give client attention without focusing specifically on physical symptoms, listen with accepting attitude to client's feelings and expressions of concern, check out that there is no organic reason for the client's physical symptoms, tell client about the availability of various psychotherapies as tools to gain insight into unconscious conflicts and/or experience support.

Exercise 6
Relieve delirium tremens in alcohol withdrawal, relieve skeletal muscle spasms, potentiate anticonvulsant medications.

Exercise 7
Personal choice.

CHAPTER 18

Exercise 1
2: Cold, unfeeling. 3: Disgust. 4: Anger. 5: Courage. 6: Insensitivity. 7: Shame, guilt, embarrassment. 8: Disgust. 9: Love. 10: Annoyance. 11: Stubbornness. 12: Pleasure, relief. 13: Indifference. 14: Curiosity, interest. 15: Fear. 16-20: Personal examples.

Exercise 2
Somatization: 2, 6, 8, 14. Conversion: 5, 9, 11, 13. Hypochondriasis: 3, 7, 12. Malingering: 1, 4, 10, 15.

Exercise 3a
Primary gains: 2, 5, 6, 7, 9. Secondary gains: 1, 3, 4, 8, 10.

Exercise 3b
Respond in a matter-of-fact manner rather than being overly sympathetic; avoid focusing on client's symptoms and making comments emphasizing secondary gains: "Now you can look at your favorite soap opera on TV every day." "You won't have to worry about that final exam in school now." "Look at all those cards! You need to get sick to see how many friends you have"; work with family, teaching them about the illness and have them help you encourage client to become autonomous; limit staff contact to those who understand and accept the client's illness; reflect on own feelings.

Exercise 4
Physical: 2: Gastrointestinal disorder in which sustained gastric hypermotility and increase in gastric secretions erode stomach lining resulting in epigastric pain 1 to 4 hours after eating. 3: Cardiovascular disorder in which there is sustained elevation of systolic and diastolic arterial blood pressure, leading to organic changes, including renal damage if condition is chronic. 4: Respiratory disorder in which bronchial obstruction interferes with expiration and results in a wheeze and leads to pulmonary changes and a decreased vital capacity. 5: Musculoskeletal disorder in which there is marked organic damage to joints as

well as other tissues. Emotional: 2: Underlying unconscious dependency needs conflict with individual's perception of himself as strong, independent, unemotional, and hard working. Illness precipitated by stress. Brings dependency-independency conflict closer to awareness. 3: Feelings of anger and rage are internalized and the individual maintains a calm, placid, compliant exterior. Tries to conform to expectations of others, demands of authority. 4: Underlying fear of abandonment by mother and mixed feelings of dependency and anger. Represses the anger. Expresses the symbolic "cry for the mother" in the asthmatic wheeze. 5: Masochistic, self-sacrificing individual with a history of maternal deprivation and unmet dependency needs.

Exercise 5b
Nursing diagnosis: Altered Gastrointestinal Processes R/T unconscious dependency-independency conflicts (ANA: 7.4.2). Nursing objectives: Physical: Help restore client's physiological homeokinesis. Emotional: Help meet client's dependency-independency needs, help reduce client's anxiety. Nursing actions: Carry out dietary modifications as prescribed, administer antacids as ordered by physician, address client as Mr. Keck, anticipate client's needs so he does not have to ask for help, seek out client and spend time with him, listen to client's concerns, tell client about availability of various psychotherapies.

Exercise 5c
Nursing diagnosis: Altered Circulation R/T repressed anger (ANA: 7.1.2). Nursing objectives: Physical: Help restore client's physiological homeokinesis. Emotional: Help client express feelings appropriately. Nursing actions: Teach client dietary management and the relationship between smoking and the development of circulatory problems, support client's efforts to give up smoking, monitor blood pressure on a regular basis, administer antihypertensive agents as ordered by the physician, encourage client to express feelings verbally, listen to client's concerns, tell client about availability of various psychotherapies.

Exercise 5d
Nursing diagnosis: Altered Oxygenation Processes R/T unconscious fear of abandonment (ANA: 7.8.2). Nursing objectives: Physical: Help restore client's physiological homeokinesis. Emotional: Help meet client's dependency needs, help reduce client's anxiety. Nursing actions: Provide bed rest during acute asthma attack, stay with client during attack, support client in sitting position during attack to facilitate breathing, give hygiene care and change bed linens after attack subsides, administer bronchodilators and expectorants as ordered by physician, listen to client's expressions of concerns, tell client about availability of various psychotherapies.

Exercise 5e
Nursing diagnosis: Altered Musculoskeletal Processes R/T conflict over unmet dependency needs and repressed anger (ANA: 7.5.2). Nursing objectives: Physical: Help restore client's physiological homeokinesis. Emotional: Help meet client's dependency needs, help client express feelings appropriately. Nursing actions: Provide bed rest, apply moist heat as ordered to the affected areas, maintain in good body alignment, provide range-of-motion exercises, administer salicylates such as aspirin as ordered by the physician, encourage expression of feelings verbally, listen to client's concerns, tell client about availability of various psychotherapies.

CHAPTER 19
Exercise 1
Personal responses.

Exercise 2
b: Hallucinatory experience resulting from impaired sensory perception is often a phenomenon noted in persons with delirium tremens. c: Substance-dependent

individuals are often manipulative and passive-aggressive. They are sometimes a source of embarrassment and fear and hence are often avoided by others. d: Levels of .05% alcohol in the blood diminish inhibitions; a person's ability to control impulses decreases as the alcohol intake increases. e: Anxiety related to inaccessibility of alcohol or drugs reflects an individual's psychological dependence on the substance (habituation). f: Individuals who use drugs and/or alcohol chronically inevitably suffer from malnutrition as they fail to consume a nutritious diet, electing to purchase drugs/alcohol instead of food. g: Excess intake of alcohol and/or drugs affects cognition, and a person's ability to make sound judgments decreases. h: Ingestion of even small amounts of LSD produces temporary hallucinations; "flashbacks" can also occur, in which the user continues to experience hallucinations days or weeks after using hallucinogens. i: Depression commonly follows withdrawal from crack and/or cocaine. If severe enough, it may even precipitate a suicide attempt. j: The individual who abuses drugs and/or alcohol has very low self-esteem, and this is reflected by an inability to meet hygiene needs.

Exercise 3a

Nursing Diagnosis #1: Nursing actions: Provide bed rest, assign client to a single room, provide quiet atmosphere and subdued lighting, provide consistency and continuity of care, administer intravenous fluids as ordered by physician, administer anticonvulsant medications and B vitamins (thiamine, niacin) as prescribed, take and record vital signs at regular intervals, institute cooling measures, call client by name and orient him to personnel and activities being carried out. Anticipated outcomes: Within 24 hours the client's physical condition will be stabilized, elevated temperature will be within normal limits, and orientation to time, place, and person returning.

Exercise 3b

Nursing Diagnosis #2: Nursing actions: Administer oral fluids, discontinue intravenous fluids as ordered, provide diet high in protein and low in fat, maintain on anticonvulsant medications and B vitamins as ordered by the physician, administer anxiolytic medications as prescribed, ambulate gradually, use side rails when client is in bed. Anticipated outcomes: Within 2 weeks the client will be ambulated, show evidence of improved nutrition, and be free of seizures. Nursing Diagnosis #3: Nursing actions: Call client by name; orient client to time, place, and person; provide consistency and continuity of care by seeking out client regularly, sitting and talking with him, and encouraging him to talk about himself and his concerns; make arrangements for his children's care and for them to visit at the hospital; support and encourage client's decision to be an active member of Alcoholics Anonymous. Anticipated outcomes: Within 2 weeks the client will be oriented to time, place, and person; be feeling more comfortable with himself; begin to attend AA meetings on a regular basis; and be discharged from the hospital.

Exercise 4

Symptoms: 2: Faulty decision making, judgment, memory; blames others for problems. 3: Neglects home environment. 4: Feels "normal" when under influence of drugs; denies having a problem; feels anxiety, guilt, shame during withdrawal. 5: Manipulates others; acts out aggressively, especially to obtain drugs; disrupts family unit; ineffective in school, on the job; alienated from people who do not use drugs. 6: Inattentive; poor self-concept. 7: Undernourished; neglects all aspects of health; prone to infection at needle sites; susceptible to acquired immune deficiency syndrome (AIDS) from contaminated needles. 8: Feelings of powerlessness, especially when not using drugs. Nursing actions: 2: Help client with decision making, such as identifying alternate choices; encourage client to look at consequences of actions. 3: Involve family resources in helping client maintain home while being treated for drug abuse. 4: Stay with client and give emotional support; encourage and listen to expressions of feelings. 5: Seek out and relate to the client; set limits on unsocialized behavior; point out consequences of undesirable behavior. 6: Seek out client and demonstrate genuine interest; call client by name; give help as necessary with appearance and hygiene; praise and give recognition for client's efforts to help self. 7: Provide nutritious diet; encourage health and dental care; teach about AIDS and how to protect self and others. 8: Listen to client's verbalization of concerns, feelings.

Exercise 5	Symptoms of narcotic withdrawal: sneezing, coryza, yawning, irritability, restlessness, abdominal cramps, vomiting, diarrhea, headache, diaphoresis, muscle and joint pain. Symptoms of alcohol withdrawal: anxiety, tremors, nausea, diaphoresis, seizures, delirium tremens.
Exercise 6a	Group experience uses group support; helps alcoholics face the reality of their alcoholism and take steps to change a life pattern; organization assists members to face life without alcohol; members are alcoholics/recovering alcoholics who have understanding and patience for each other; promotes self-esteem by seeking out alcoholics, encouraging their attendance at AA meetings, helping them find jobs.
Exercise 6b	Advantages: Provide more humane withdrawal; halts criminal activities; increases potential for self-support; increases individual's ability to function; fairly inexpensive; fairly successful. Disadvantages: Synthetic narcotic; maintains addiction; unless highly motivated to give up addiction, individual often returns to it after treatment.

CHAPTER 20

Exercise 1	Personal responses.
Exercise 2	Behaviors: 2: Poor judgment and decision making; personalized interpretation of actions of others. 3: Not applicable. 4: Extreme mood swings from depths of depression to elation, plus feelings of anger and anxiety. 5: Intense but superficial and short-term relationships; strained family, work, and school relationships. 6: Faulty self-perception; mimicking behavior in which idealized behaviors are temporarily internalized. 7: Self-destructive behaviors: suicidal gestures, neglect of nutrition and injuries, leading to infection. 8: Unclear value system. Nursing actions: 2: Use contract to identify goals and activities to be carried out in the nurse-client relationship. 3: Not applicable. 4: Label and discuss feelings being experienced; identify themes and patterns that perpetuate various emotions. 5: Enforce consistent limits on behavior; avoid attempts to be manipulated. 6: Acceptance; consistent communication of value and worth. 7: Prevent and/or intervene in suicide attempts; provide well-balanced diet; treat injuries, infections. 8: Allow and encourage discussion of feelings of guilt and remorse for behaviors in conflict with value system.
Exercise 3a	Cognitive: 1, 3, 6, 7, 9, 10, 11. Relationships: 1, 4, 9, 10, 14. Insight/Judgment: 2, 3, 6, 9, 11, 12, 13. Impulses: 2, 3, 5, 7, 10, 12, 13. Identification: 3, 4, 8, 15.
Exercise 3b	Nursing actions: Set firm, reasonable, consistent limits and controls on behaviors; provide structured, controlled environment; hold client to the terms of the contract and his obligations; direct client's energies into challenging daily activities; reward acceptable behavior. Outcome criteria: Within two weeks the client will begin to accept limits placed on impulsive acts; follow established routine; follow through on obligations and responsibilities; participate in daily activities.

CHAPTER 21

Exercise 1
Life review: 1, 5, 12. Loneliness: 7, 10. Depression: 6, 11, 15. Suspicion: 3, 9. Dementia: 2, 8, 14. Loss: 4, 13.

Exercise 2a
Hints of despair: "I look at the future, I shudder with dread," balanced with hope: "But inside this old carcass a young girl still dwells, and now and again my battered heart swells," and acceptance with integrity: "And accept the stark fact that nothing can last."

Exercise 2b
The nurse does not talk or share her thoughts with the client; she uses a loud voice unnecessarily and fails to check if client can hear; scolds, gives disapproval rather than acknowledge client's efforts to help and does not allow client to do what she can for herself, promoting unnecessary dependency.

Exercise 2c
"A crabbit old woman, not very wise"; "Who dribbles her food, and makes no reply"; "Who seems not to notice the things that you do"; "And forever is losing a stocking or shoe"; "Who . . . lets you do as you will with bathing and feeding."

Exercise 2d
1: Have the same nurses work with the client; set up a routine that is predictable; surround client with familiar objects; provide client with hearing aid and glasses as needed; orient the client; be consistent. 2: Orient client; use her name; use touch to make contact; provide adequate light, including a dim night light; provide hearing aid and eyeglasses as needed; have patience. 3: Acknowledge pain associated with loss; use a variety of communication skills to help client focus on and express feelings; listen; use touch to make contact and communicate understanding and reassurance. 4: Develop nurse-client relationship; spend short periods with client regularly rather than long periods irregularly; ambulate client and promote socialization with other clients by having client sit in community areas and eat in dining room rather than stay alone in own room. 5: Communicate respect by calling client by surname; help with hygiene and appearance as needed; give positive feedback when appropriate; listen with interest to client's conversations; be alert to suicidal ideation. 6: Encourage client to talk about the past; allow client to keep mementoes from the past; listen when client talks about the future, death, etc.

Exercise 3
b: Elderly persons, especially those with physical illness, may experience depression and despair and see no alternative except death. They fear pain, loneliness, the process of dying, and lack of control and may attempt suicide. c: The elderly tend to focus on the past and seem to have difficulty recalling recent events. The life review, in which they reminisce, focuses on the past as a way of resolving past crises and achieving closure to one's life. d: Elderly clients who are aware of loss of mental acuity experience feelings of helplessness and hopelessness, feelings basic to the development of low self-esteem. e: Individuals with Alzheimer's disease become increasingly unable to meet their hygiene and self-care needs, primarily because of memory loss in which they forget to carry out basic care. f: Elderly persons who had difficulty mastering the task of trust in their developmental years are particularly susceptible to developing feelings of suspiciousness in their later years if they also experience visual and hearing impairment. Sensory deficits interfere with the client's ability to check out reality, and there may be a tendency to distort the innocent actions of others, based on their inherent lack of trust.

Exercise 4
Behaviors: 2: Impaired decision making, judgment, knowledge, learning, memory, etc. 3: Increasingly unable to care for own home. 4: Depression and anger early in the disorder, mood swings later. 5: Social isolation and withdrawal. 6: Increasingly distractible; aware they are having difficulty concentrating with re-

sultant loss of self-esteem. 7: Incontinence, seizures, injuries, poor hygiene and nutrition, infections. 8: Helplessness, hopelessness, powerlessness, spiritual distress. Nursing actions: 2: Use communication skills, sensory stimulation, life review, individually and in groups to stimulate discussion of ideas, expression of feelings. 3: Assist client to continue routine tasks for as long as possible; install environmental safety measures. 4: Provide opportunities for discussion of feelings early in disease process; observe for suicidal ideation; prevent suicide attempts. 5: Seek out client; encourage one-to-one and group relationships; use clear and consistent communication. 6: Accept client and respond nonjudgmentally; call client by name; treat with respect and dignity. 7: Protect from injury, seizures; maintain hygiene and nutrition; provide physical care as need arises. 8: Listen to the client.

CHAPTER 22

Exercise 1 Personal responses.

Exercise 2 Mental retardation is the term used to describe a condition in which the individual's intellectual, cognitive, and social development is delayed during the formative years of life.

Exercise 3 Degree of severity: 1: Mild. 2: Moderate. 3: Severe. 4: Profound. Characteristics: 1: Can benefit from some academic training, learn social adjustment, and have vocational preparation which allows them to be employed in simple, repetitive jobs. Able to live independently with support services. 2: Can learn to talk, master sufficient skills so that they can meet basic needs with supervision. Can function fairly well and are employable in unskilled jobs. 3: Some individuals can learn to talk and be trained in basic hygiene skills. 4: Too retarded to benefit from even simple educational programs. Require extensive care and protection against physical injury.

Exercise 4 1: Potential for Violence: Directed at others R/T poor impulse control (NANDA:9.2.2). 2: Substance Abuse R/T anger at mother (ANA:5.3.2.8), Anxiety R/T use of LSD (NANDA:9.3.1). 3: Altered Health Maintenance R/T binge and purge episodes (ANA:1.3.4.4; NANDA:6.4.2). 4: Altered Hygiene R/T severe cognitive deficit (ANA:1.3.4.6), Bathing/Hygiene Self Care Deficit R/T severe cognitive deficit (NANDA:6.5.2). 5: Potential for Violence: Self Directed R/T low self esteem and feelings of failure (ANA:5.3.1.1; NANDA:9.2.2). 6: Compulsive Behaviors R/T low self esteem (ANA:5.7.2.2), Impaired Home Maintenance Management R/T preoccupation with cleanliness (NANDA:6.4.1.1). 7: Altered Social Interaction R/T fear of relating (ANA:5.7.2). Impaired Social Interaction R/T fear of relating (NANDA:3.1.1). 8: Social Isolation/Withdrawal R/T brain dysfunction (ANA:5.7.2.5), Social Isolation R/T brain dysfunction (NANDA:3.1.2).

Exercise 5a 1: Provide firm, supportive, consistent, understanding, collaborative approach by staff; intravenous fluids; balanced diet; dietary supplements and vitamins as ordered; allow client to eat in private; routine weighing; limit exercise routine. 2: Involve client in the treatment plans; hygiene care; give deserved praise and compliments for weight gain and improved appearance; encourage peer contacts; focus on client's interests and feelings; listen; be alert to cues of suicidal ideation; refer for psychotherapy.

Exercise 5b 1: Provide firm, supportive, consistent, understanding, collaborative approach by staff; balanced diet; supervise bathroom activities to prevent self-induced vomiting; restrict use of laxatives; routine but supervised weighing schedule. 2: Develop therapeutic nurse-client relationship; show acceptance and understanding; involve client in treatment plans; hygiene care; give deserved praise and recognition for adhering to plan of care; encourage expressions of feelings; be alert to cues of suicidal ideation; refer for psychotherapy, group therapy.

CHAPTER 23	
Exercise 1	Personal responses.
Exercise 2	b: Seriously ill persons realize that without the transplant they will probably die in a short time and, also, failure of the transplanted organ to be accepted by the body can also result in death. c: Persons who lose a body part often experience a changed body image and go through a period of grief and mourning. d: A characteristic response to cardiac surgery for persons with long-term cardiac pathology is anger over the dependency role coupled with the anticipation and hope that they will be able to lead more normal, autonomous lives. e: Women who give birth to defective infants often feel responsible, guilty, question their own value as women, and experience loss of self-esteem. f: Women who terminate an unwanted pregnancy, a pregnancy resulting from rape or incest, or a pregnancy in which a severe genetic defect has been identified experience conflict with society's attitudes and values concerning abortion and the *right to life*. g: Individuals with AIDS are often stigmatized and rejected by family, friends, and society because of the individuals' life-style and because these people fear infection by the AIDS virus. At the same time, the AIDS victim withdraws in fear of transmitting the virus to others.
Exercise 3	Provide good physical care; anticipate needs before client has to ask; use an unhurried approach; listen to expressions of anger and resentment without getting angry or defensive in return; avoid use of meaningless cliches in an attempt to reassure or minimize concerns; explain tests, procedures, and answer questions; spend time with client; involve client in planning care; acknowledge and include family in care.
Exercise 4a	a: 10, 11. b: 2, 19, 25. c: 3, 6, 9, 24, 27, 28, 32, 35. d: 3, 8, 21, 34. e: 7, 14, 31, 34, 36, 37. f: 5, 11, 12, 17, 18, 20, 23, 29. g: 1, 15, 16. h: 13, 22, 32, 33. i: 4, 5, 12, 17, 23, 24, 26, 30.
Exercise 4b	Characteristics: 1: Person is unable to deal with reality of her impending death. Uses ego defense to defend. 2: Person experiences anger, resentment; feels she is the victim of fate, circumstances, incompetence of others, etc. 3: Individual attempts to bargain or trade off "good" behavior for more time. 4: Individual is no longer able to avoid reality of impending death and is aware that denial, anger, and bargaining are ineffective. Respond to anticipated loss with depression. 5: Person comes to peace with herself about fact she is dying. Characterized by "affective void"—she is neither happy nor depressed. Interests are limited. Behaviors: 1: Not wanting to talk about fears; "Why borrow trouble?"; trying to put fears out of mind (suppression). 2: Verbal expressions of anger directed at nurse; nonverbal anger, tense posture, frown, etc. 3: Identifying herself as not very cooperative; offers to try to be "good"; hoping to live long enough to see daughter grow up, get settled. 4: Lying in the dark; alone; not eating; giving up— "What's the use?," "Beginning of the end." "Time I faced the truth." 5: Sense of completion—has finished the diary, the painting; taking pleasure in accomplishments; talks about dying more easily; limited interests—mainly concerned about being free of pain.

CHAPTER 24

Exercise 1 "Mental health authorities define a crisis as a state of disequilibrium resulting from the interaction of an event with the individual's or family's coping mechanisms, which are inadequate to meet the demands of the situation, combined with the individual's or family's perception of the meaning of the event." (Taylor, Chapter 24)

Exercise 2 Developmental: 1, 2, 3, 5, 6, 8, 14. Situational: 4, 7, 9, 10, 11, 12, 13, 15.

Exercise 3 Massive amounts of free-floating anxiety; self-limiting; highly individual threat; affects significant others in the individual's support system.

Exercise 4 Denial: 1, 6, 7. Increased tension: 5, 12. Disorganization: 3, 8, 11. Reorganization: 2, 9. Escape the problem: 4, 10.

Exercise 5 a: 13, 17, 19, 23. b: 3, 6, 7, 14, 21, 26, 27, 29, 31. c: 10, 32, 35. d: 1, 2, 21, 25, 28. e: 9, 15, 20, 30. f: 5, 12, 20, 40. g: 8, 34. h: 3, 6, 7, 27, 29, 31. i: 15, 22, 24, 36, 39. j: 4, 5, 11, 16, 18, 33, 37, 38.

CHAPTER 25

Exercise 1 1: Membership. 2: Subgroups. 3: Goals. 4: Roles. 5: Norms. 6: Identity. 7: Attractiveness. 8: Phases.

Exercise 2 a: Jason; b: Helen; c: Kirby; d: Paula; e: Rob; f: Carol; g: Tom; h: Arthur.

Exercise 3 Preaffiliation: 1, 8, 12, 13. Intragroup conflict: 3, 5, 9, 15. Working: 4, 6, 7, 14. Termination: 2, 10, 11.

Exercise 4 Therapy: 1, 4, 5, 6, 7, 9, 10, 13. Socialization: 2, 3, 8, 11, 12, 14, 15.

CHAPTER 26

Exercise 1 Regulation of sexual activity and reproduction; physical maintenance; protection; education and socialization; recreation; conferring of status; giving of affection.

Exercise 2 Onset: Stage I, Phase 2: Begins with wife's pregnancy. Stage II: Begins with birth of first child. Stage III: Begins when the eldest child enters school. Stage IV: Begins when the eldest child becomes an adolescent. Stage V: Begins when the children are preparing to or are actually leaving home. Stage VI: Begins when all the children have left home and there are no children to parent. Stage VII: Begins with retirement. Goal: Stage I, Phase 2: To adjust to wife's pregnancy. Stage II: To meet needs of infants and preschool children. Stage III: To protect school-aged children from undesirable influences outside the home while enabling them to fit into the world. Stage IV: To loosen family ties to permit greater freedom and responsibility for the members. Stage V: To release its members to assume adult responsibilities. Stage VI: To maintain marital relationships. Stage VII: To prepare for dissolution of the family. Family dynamics: Stage I, Phase 2: Wife becomes self-absorbed as she prepares for the birth; husband generally feels increased responsibility. Stage II: Roles of husband and wife expand to include those of father and mother. Stage III: Composition of family may include preschool children as well as school-aged children; the latter need support to deal with societal values that may conflict with family values. Stage IV: Children may overreact to greater freedom causing parents to respond with more rather than less control. Stage V: The "launching stage" in which parents and children all experience difficulty with releasing members and assuming adult responsibility. Stage VI: The "postparental family" in which parents subsume their parental roles into their marital roles; experience the "empty nest" syndrome. Stage VII: The retirement and postretirement years in which the couple prepares for dissolution of the family by death of one of the spouses.

Exercise 3	Blended family: 2, 5, 10, 19. Extended family: 3, 11, 14, 18. Household concept: 7, 9, 13, 16, 17, 20. Nuclear family: 1, 4, 6, 8, 12, 15.
Exercise 4	Effective: 1, 2, 5, 6, 8, 10, 14, 15. Ineffective: 3, 4, 7, 9, 11, 12, 13.
Exercise 5	See Taylor, Chapter 26, Table 26-1 for a complete listing of physical and behavioral indicators of child abuse and neglect.
Exercise 6	To resolve pathological conflicts and anxiety within the family; to strengthen the individual member against destructive forces within him/herself and within the family; to strengthen the family against critical upsets; to influence the orientation of the family identity; to promote a value of health in the family.

Answers to test items

Chapter 1   1-a 2-a 3-d 4-d 5-b 6-c 7-a 8-c 9-d 10-b 11-b 12-d 13-c 14-b 15-b 16-d 17-a 18-d 19-b 20-d 21-d 22-a 23-d 24-a 25-a

Chapter 2   1-b 2-c 3-d 4-b 5-b 6-d 7-b 8-c 9-d 10-d 11-a 12-b 13-d 14-a 15-a

Chapter 3   1-d 2-c 3-b 4-a 5-b 6-d 7-c 8-d 9-c 10-b 11-d 12-a 13-a 14-c 15-b

Chapter 4   1-c 2-a 3-b 4-b 5-c 6-d 7-a 8-d 9-b 10-a 11-d 12-a 13-d 14-b 15-d

Chapter 5   1-d 2-c 3-d 4-b 5-b 6-a 7-b 8-c 9-b 10-d 11-a 12-a 13-b 14-c 15-d

Chapter 6   1-a 2-c 3-c 4-b 5-b 6-a 7-d 8-d 9-c 10-d 11-b 12-c 13-d 14-d 15-b 16-b 17-a 18-b 19-a 20-c 21-b 22-a 23-b 24-b 25-d

Chapter 7   1-b 2-b 3-d 4-d 5-c 6-a 7-d 8-c 9-a 10-c 11-a 12-b 13-d 14-c 15-b 16-b 17-c 18-a 19-c 20-b 21-a 22-d 23-b 24-c- 25-c

Chapter 8   1-a 2-d 3-c 4-b 5-d 6-d 7-c 8-d 9-b 10-b 11-a 12-b 13-b 14-c 15-b

Chapter 9   1-a 2-d 3-b 4-d 5-c 6-d 7-a 8-a 9-a 10-c 11-c 12-a 13-d 14-b 15-d 16-c 17-b 18-b 19-c 20-b 21-c 22-b 23-d 24-d 25-d

Chapter 10   1-c 2-d 3-b 4-a 5-d 6-d 7-d 8-a 9-b 10-d 11-c 12-c 13-b 14-a 15-a

Chapter 11   1-c 2-b 3-d 4-a 5-b 6-a 7-d 8-a 9-b 10-a 11-d 12-a 13-c 14-b 15-b 16-a 17-c 18-d 19-a 20-b 21-b 22-d 23-b 24-b 25-d

Chapter 12   1-a 2-b 3-b 4-d 5-c 6-a 7-c 8-a 9-c 10-b 11-d 12-d 13-b 14-d 15-c 16-d 17-c 18-a 19-a 20-c

Chapter 13   1-b 2-c 3-a 4-d 5-a 6-d 7-c 8-a 9-b 10-a 11-d 12-c 13-c 14-d 15-d

Chapter 14   1-c 2-b 3-d 4-c 5-d 6-d 7-c 8-a 9-b 10-d 11-a 12-d 13-b 14-a 15-d

Chapter 15   1-a 2-c 3-c 4-a 5-d 6-b 7-b 8-d 9-a 10-d 11-c 12-b 13-b 14-d 15-b 16-c 17-d 18-c 19-a 20-a 21-c 22-d 23-c 24-c 25-a

Chapter 16   1-a 2-d 3-a 4-b 5-c 6-c 7-d 8-c 9-c 10-d 11-b 12-a 13-d 14-d 15-a 16-b 17-b 18-d 19-c 20-a 21-b 22-b 23-c 24-a 25-a

Chapter 17   1-a 2-c 3-c 4-d 5-a 6-b 7-d 8-c 9-d 10-a 11-d 12-a 13-a 14-d 15-b 16-c 17-b 18-d 19-a 20-b

Chapter 18   1-d 2-d 3-b 4-a 5-c 6-a 7-d 8-c 9-a 10-a 11-d 12-a 13-c 14-d 15-a 16-b 17-d 18-a 19-c 20-a

Chapter 19 1-a 2-d 3-d 4-b 5-c 6-b 7-b 8-a 9-d 10-c 11-d 12-b 13-a 14-c 15-a 16-b 17-c 18-c 19-b 20-a

Chapter 20 1-a 2-d 3-d 4-b 5-d 6-c 7-b 8-a 9-d 10-a 11-b 12-a 13-c 14-d 15-c

Chapter 21 1-d 2-a 3-c 4-b 5-d 6-a 7-b 8-c 9-d 10-b 11-d 12-b 13-c 14-b 15-d

Chapter 22 1-a 2-b 3-b 4-d 5-d 6-c 7-a 8-d 9-b 10-c 11-b 12-d 13-a 14-b 15-c 16-b 17-d 18-d 19-c 20-c

Chapter 23 1-c 2-d 3-d 4-b 5-a 6-a 7-b 8-d 9-c 10-d 11-b 12-d 13-c 14-b 15-c

Chapter 24 1-b 2-b 3-c 4-c 5-a 6-b 7-a 8-d 9-a 10-c 11-c 12-b 13-a 14-d 15-d

Chapter 25 1-a 2-d 3-b 4-c 5-d 6-c 7-a 8-a 9-d 10-a 11-b 12-c 13-b 14-d 15-d

Chapter 26 1-c 2-b 3-c 4-a 5-d 6-b 7-c 8-b 9-a 10-d 11-b 12-a 13-d 14-c 15-b

Solutions to word games and section exercises

MATCHING

Section one
2-Rush, 3-Beers, 4-Kennedy, 5-Tracy, 6-Freud, 7-Pinel, 8-Mitchell, 9-Dix, 10-Jarrett.

Section two
1-Render, 2-Freud, 3-Jones, 4-Luft, 5-Peplau, 6-Ruesch.

Section three
2-Erikson, 3-Szasz, 4-Jahoda, 5-Selye, 6-Kallman, 7-Horney, 8-von Bertalanffy, 9-Freud, 10-Becker, 11-Piaget, 12-Sullivan, 13-Carlson, 14-Charcot, 15-Maslow.

Section four
a   Historical perspective: 2-Kubler-Ross, 3-Cerletti, 4-Kernberg, 5-Bleuler, 6-Alzheimer, 7-Alexander, 8-Sakel, 9-Moustakos, 10-Krapelin.
b   Psychotropic medications: 1-Thorazine, 2-Mellaril, 3-Quide, 4-Serentil, 5-Prolixin, 6-Trilafon, 7-Stelazine, 8-Haldol, 9-Taractan, 10-Navane, 11-Moban, 12-Loxitane, 13-Tofranil, 14-Elavil, 15-Pertofrane, 16-Norpramin, 17-Aventyl, 18-Pamelor, 19-Sinequan, 20-Adapin, 21-Marplan, 22-Nardil, 23-Parnate, 28-Valium, 29-Xanax, 30-Librium, 31-Tranxene, 32-Paxipam, 33-Ativan, 34-Serax, 35-Centrax.

Section five
2-Feldman, 3-Satir, 4-Perls, 5-Menninger, 6-Bales, 7-Ackerman, 8-Caplan, 9-Duvall, 10-Berne.

LOGIC

Section one
Client Rights: Treatment-Chin-Todd, Habeus Corpus-Williams-Eddy, Confidentiality-Solo-May, Informed Consent-Ames-Mac, Least Restrictive Treatment-Low-Cobb.

Section five
Therapies: Bette-Family-Monday, Lawrence-Conjoint-Friday, Dexter-Gestalt-Wednesday, Frank-Psychodrama-Thursday, Janet-TA-Tuesday.

FILL-IN

Section two
Nursing interactions: A-principles, B-double bind, C-rapport, D-counselor, E-milieu, F-intervention, G-suggesting, H-limit setting, I-maintenance, J-introspection, K-emergency, L-recording, M-goal, N-outcomes, O-emotions, P-client, Q-exploring, R-signs, S-assessment.

Section three
Mental mechanisms: A-sublimation, B-conversion, C-undoing, D-fixation, E-isolation, F-denial, G-problem solving, H-regression, I-preoccupation, J-apathy, K-displacement, L-rationalization, M-symbolization, N-suppression, O-compensation, P-repression.

6 × 6: Feelings

Section two
Anger, apathy, awe, doom, fear, glee, gloom, grief, guilt, hate, ire, joy, love, pain, panic, pity, rage, regret, relief, woe.

QUOTE-A-CROSTIC

Section two

Nurse–Peggy Anderson. "I love to think about what goes on in people's minds. I love to watch their eyes and watch the way they react to things . . . I've learned a lot from patients about human beings." (New York, Berkley Publishing Corp., 1979, p. 41.)

A-nonverbal
B-thank you
C-therapist
D-beliefs, attitudes
E-aye
F-problem solving
G-state
H-teaching
I-agent
J-empathy
K-who, what
L-one-to-one
M-data
N-theme
O-revision
P-holistic
Q-touch
R-Window

Section three

Second Heaven–Judith Guest. "Nearly all her life she had read for escape . . . newspapers, magazines, bad novels, good novels, billboard signs, cereal boxes. She read all her junk mail, putting words, tons of words, between her and the thing that had happened to her." (New York, New American Library, A Signet Book, 1983, pp. 82-83.)

A-stress
B-labeled
C-phallic phase
D-mood
E-anal zone
F-feedback
G-endorphin
H-power
I-lead
J-deviant behavior
K-wellness
L-warn
M-Jahoda
N-shame and doubt
O-DNA
P-interpersonal theory
Q-fight-or-flight
R-baths
S-regress
T-laugh
U-gender
V-wholeness
W-experts

Section four

Personhood–Leo F. Buscaglia. "Most people abhor the very idea of pain . . . They seek to evade it . . . They perform all types of mental gymnastics . . . or blind themselves with momentary sources of relief such as alcohol, tranquilizers and drugs. Some, in desperation, will even choose psychosis . . ." (New York, Fawcett Columbine, 1982, p. 123.)

A-symptom
B-hysteria
C-mother
D-dysfunction
E-quiet room
F-loneliness
G-myth
H-adaptation
I-orders
J-SAD
K-powerlessness
L-hooked
M-sobs
N-affect
O-bereavement
P-Fluid Volume
Q-notes
R-schizophrenia
S-hyperactive
T-Physiological Processes
U-mental health
V-life review
W-allergy

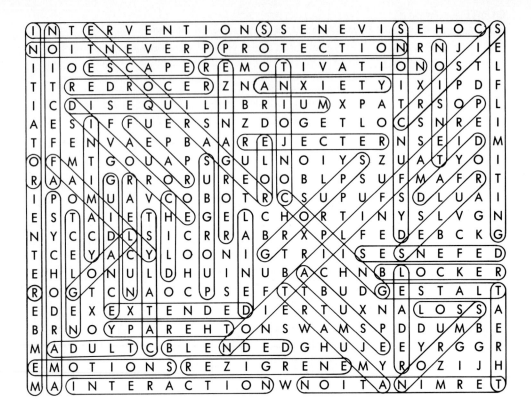

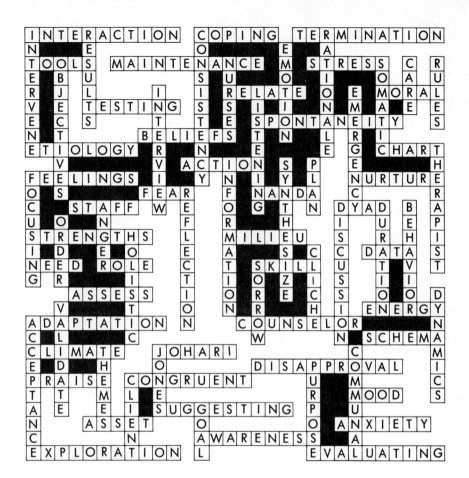

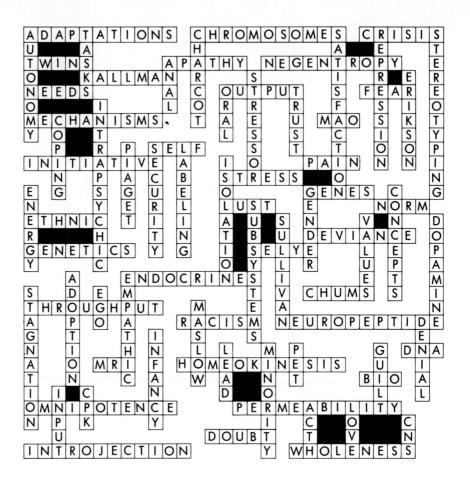

Section four

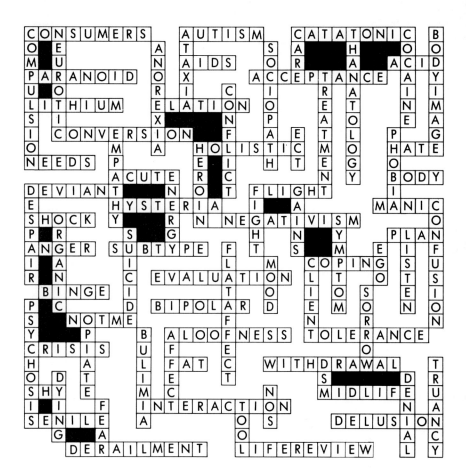

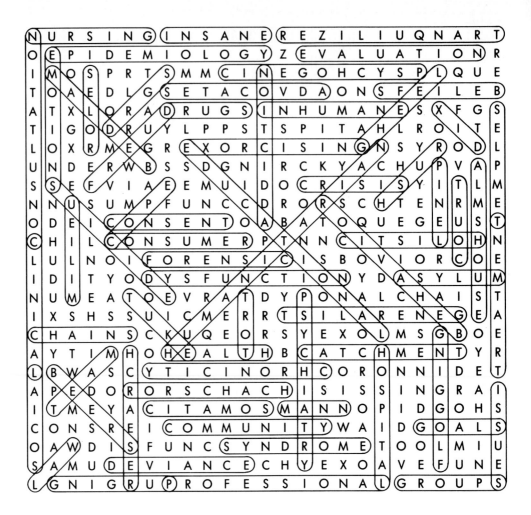

Index

A

Abortion, attitudes towards client considering, 209, 219-220

Abuse
 child, 254
 drug and alcohol; *see* Substance abuse and dependence

Acceptance, 43-44, 222
 stage of dying, 225-226

Activity therapist, 4

Adaptation
 stress and, 78, 79

Admission, psychiatric, 8, 9

Adolescents with dysfunctional behaviors, 207-217
 attitudes towards, 208-209

Affect
 flat, 123
 inappropriate, 119, 123

Affective disorders; *see* Mania; Depression

Aging; *see* Elderly

Alcohol dependence; *see* Substance abuse and dependence

Alcoholics Anonymous, 180, 184-185, 187

Alzheimer's disease, nursing actions associated with behaviors in, 204

Ambivalence, 119, 123

ANA Classification of Human Response Patterns, 60, 62, 126, 140-143, 156-159, 171-175, 181-183, 184-185, 186, 193, 194, 203, 204, 211-212, 213-214, 220-221

Anorexia nervosa
 attitudes towards client with, 208-209
 care plan for client with, 213-214
 nursing diagnosis for client with, 211-212

Antianxiety agents, 160-161

Anticipatory grieving, care plan for client experiencing, 140

Antidepressant medications, 143-145, 231

Antimanic medications, 143, 146, 231

Antipsychotic medications, 128-130, 230

Antisocial behavior; *see* Personality disorders

Anxiety, 94-100
 anxiolytic medications and, 160-161

Anxiety—cont'd
 intrapsychic vs. interpersonal theory, 94-95
 levels of, 94
 mental mechanisms and, 98
 self awareness and, 96-97

Anxiety disorders, 150-163
 anxiolytic medications and, 160-161
 care plans for clients with, 156-159
 defense mechanisms and, 151, 154-155
 intrapsychic theory and, 150-151, 152-153
 symptomatology reflecting, 156

Anxiolytic medications, 160-161, 231

Apathy, 98
 mental mechanism, 95, 98
 symptom of schizophrenia, 119

Appraisals, reflected, 87-88, 89, 97

Approach; *see* Nursing approaches

Assessment; *see* Nursing process

Associative looseness, 119, 123

Attitudes towards
 adolescents and children with dysfunctional behavior, 208-209
 clients with AIDS, 220
 mentally ill persons, 23-24
 persons with personality disorders, 191-192
 physically ill individuals, 219-220
 substance abusers, 179-180, 180-181

Auditory hallucinations, 123

Autism, 123
 attitudes towards children exhibiting, 208-209
 nursing diagnosis for children with, 211-212

Autistic thinking, 119

Autoimmune deficiency syndrome (AIDS), 179
 attitudes towards client with, 220

Awareness, self-; *see* Self-assessment

B

Bad-me, 87-88, 89

Bargaining, 224-225, 226

Behaviors associated with,
 alcohol withdrawal, 187
 Alzheimer's disease, 204
 anxiety disorders, 154-155, 156